LOW-CARB RECIPES

Side Dish Salad

Beef

Hot Vegetable Dishes

The Complete Guide With Simple and Yummy Low-Carb Recipes to Impress Your Friends And Family

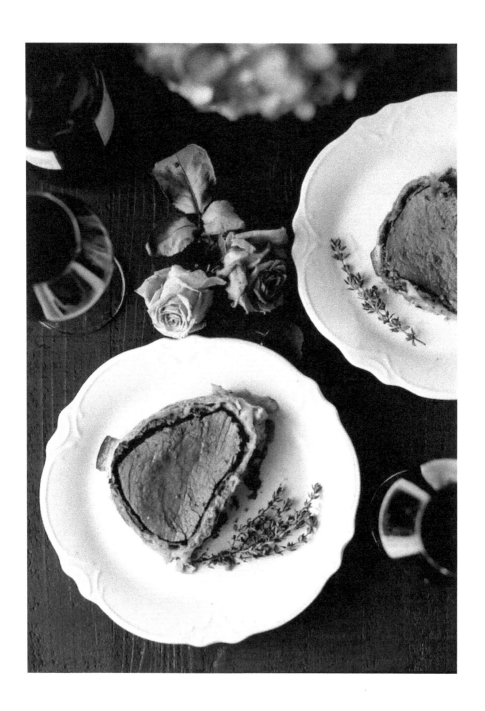

Beef

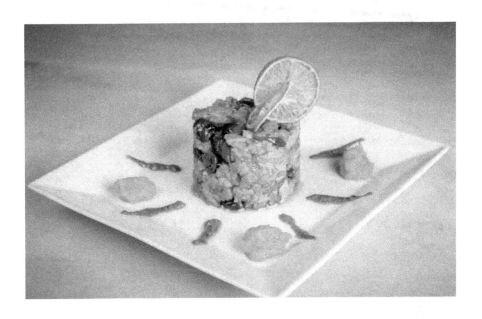

There seems to be no end to the ways we can use beef-by itself, in casseroles, and in sandwiches, sauces, and pizzas, beef is a delicious way to get plenty of protein for no carbs at all.

This chapter gives you some low-carb editions of high-carb favorites, as well as showing you some ways to use beef that you may never have even considered before. So read on.

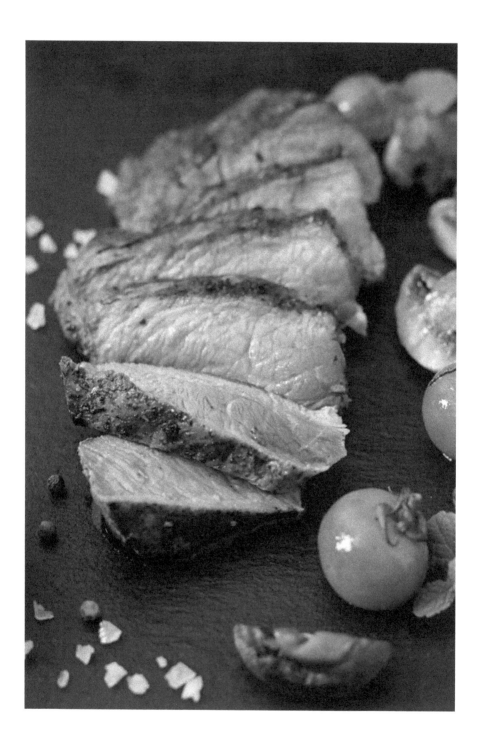

Hamburgers

Let's talk about hamburgers for a moment.
There is much to be said in favor of he
humble hamburger-it's cheap, it's quick, it's
easy, and just about everybody likes it.
Rarely will you hear the kids complain, "Oh,
no. Hamburgers again?"
Furthermore, it's a food that is easy to make
for both the "normal" eaters and the low-
carbers: Just leave the bun off of yours!
On the other hand, plain hamburgers,
without a bun, can become just a wee bit
boring to the adult palate over time. What
follows are some recipes to help you vary
your burgers. All the carb and protein
analyses are based on burgers
that weigh 1/3 pound before cooking.

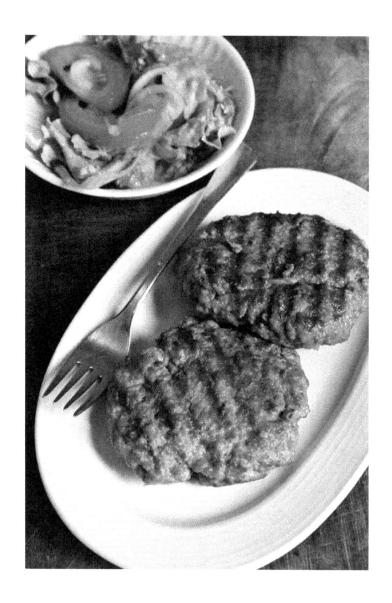

Bleu Burger

1 hamburger patty
1 tablespoon crumbled blue cheese
1 teaspoon finely minced sweet red onion

Cook your burger by your preferred method. When it's almost done to your liking, top with the bleu cheese and let it melt. Remove from the heat, put it on plate, and top with onion.

Yield: 1 serving, with only a trace of carbohydrates,
no fiber, and 27 grams
of protein.

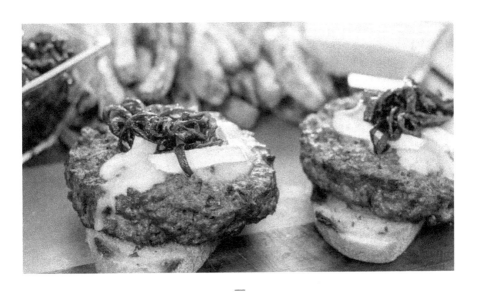

Smothered Burgers

Mmmmushrooms and onions!

4 hamburger patties
2 tablespoons butter or olive oil
1/2 cup sliced onion
1/2 cup sliced mushrooms
Dash of Worcestershire sauce

Cook your burgers by your preferred method. While the burgers are cooking, melt the butter or heat the oil in a small, heavy skillet over medium-high heat. Add the onion and mushrooms, and saute until the onions are translucent. Add a dash of Worcestershire sauce, stir, and spoon over burgers.

Yield: 4 servings, each with just 2 grams of carbohydrates, at least a trace of fiber,
and 27 grams of protein.

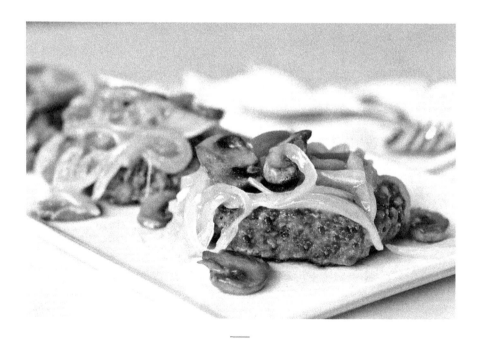

Mexiburgers

1 hamburger patty
1 ounce jalepeno Jack or Monterey Jack cheese
1 tablespoon salsa

Cook your burger by your preferred method. When it's almost done to your liking, melt the cheese over the burger. Top with salsa and serve.

Yield: 1 serving, with 2 grams of carbohydrates, a trace of fiber, and 27 grams of
protein.

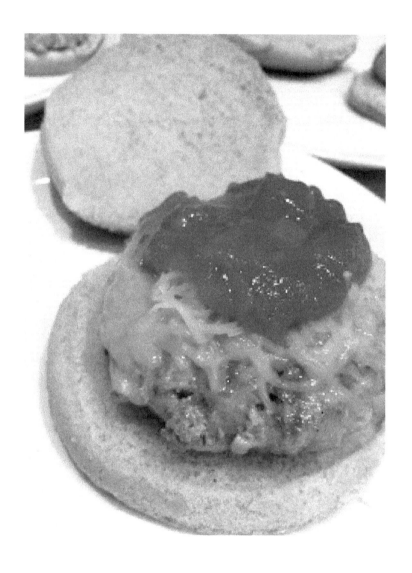

Poor Man's Poivrade

A real peppery bite-not for the timid!
1 hamburger patty
1 tablespoon coarse cracked pepper
1 tablespoon butter
2 tablespoons dry white wine, dry sherry, or dry vermouth

1. Roll your raw hamburger patty in the pepper until it's coated allover.
2. Fry the burger in the butter over medium heat, until it's done to your liking.
3. Remove the burger to a plate. Add the wine to the skillet, and stir it around for a minute or two, until all the nice brown crusty bits are scraped up. Pour this over the hamburger, and serve.

Yield: 1 serving, with between 4 and 6 grams of
carbohydrates per serving
(depending on whether you use wine, sherry, or vermouth-
wine is lowest,
vermouth is highest) and 2 grams of fiber, for a total of 2 to 4
grams of usable
carbs and 27 grams of protein.

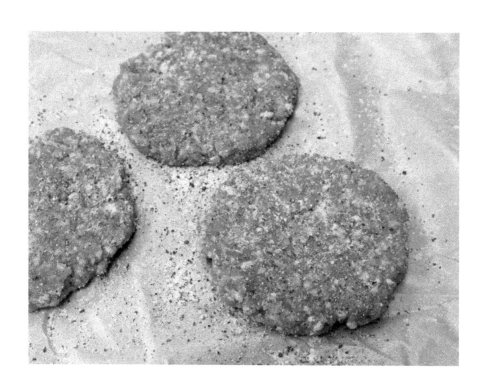

Pizza Burger

1 hamburger patty
1 tablespoon sugar-free jarred pizza sauce
2 tablespoons shredded mozzarella cheese

Cook the burger by your preferred method. When it's almost done to your liking, top with pizza sauce, then mozzarella. Cook until the cheese is melted, and serve.

Yield: 1 serving, with (depending on your brand of pizza sauce), no more than 2
grams of carbohydrates, no fiber, and 28 grams of protein.

~ One of the lowest-carb nationally distributed brands of spaghetti sauce is
Hunt's Classic. It has 7.5 grams of carbs per 1/2-CUp serving, of which 4 g is
fiber, for an effective carb count of just 3.5 grams.

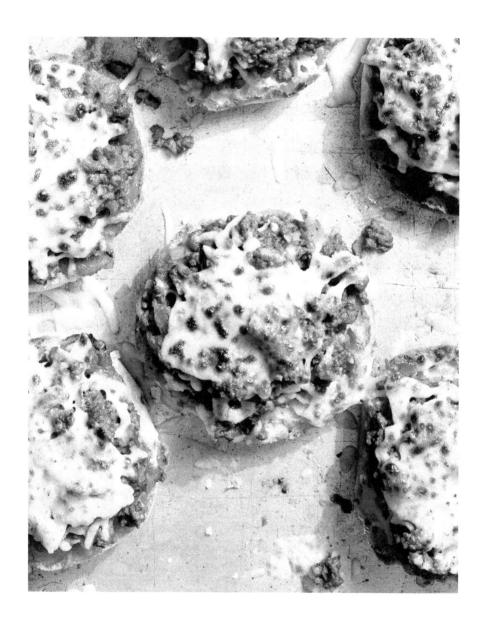

Ellen's Noodleless Lasagne

Ellen Radke sent this recipe for all you folks who miss lasagne! My dear friend Maria, who tested it on her husband and five kids, was asked if she would make this again. Her answer? An enthusiastic "Yes!"

1 pound ground beef
1 cup low-carb spaghetti sauce
1 can (4 ounces) sliced mushrooms
1 cup ricotta cheese
1 egg, beaten
1 1/2 cups shredded mozzarella cheese
1/2 tablespoon Italian seasoning
20 to 25 slices pepperoni

1. Preheat the oven to 350°F.
2. Brown the ground beef in a frying pan, and drain off the oil. Add the spaghetti sauce and mushrooms, and simmer 10 minutes.
3. In a small bowl, mix the ricotta, egg, 1/4 cup mozzarella, and Italian seasoning. Beat well with a fork.
4. Grease an 8 x 8-inch glass baking dish with nonstick cooking spray. Spread the beef mixture in the bottom of the dish. Spread the ricotta mixture on top of the beef mixture. Lay half the pepperoni slices on top of the ricotta mixture. Put remaining 1 cup of the shredded mozzarella over the pepperoni slices, and lay the remaining pepperoni on top of the cheese. Bake until bubbly (about 20 minutes).

Yield: 4 servings, each with 9 grams of carbohydrates and 3 grams of fiber, for a
total of 6 grams of usable carbs and 43 grams of protein.
~ Recipe-tester Ellen adds: "Next time, I'll try mixing in some Parmesan
cheese with the ricotta, and maybe adding a layer of spinach."

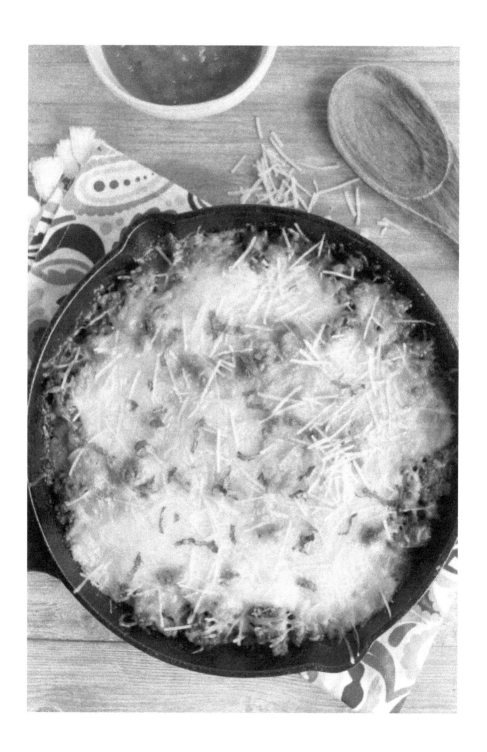

Ultra Meat Sauce

Spaghetti without the spaghetti, as it were.

1 1/2 pounds of ground beef
1 small onion, diced
1 clove garlic crushed
1 green pepper, diced
1 can (4 ounces) mushrooms, drained
2 cups low-carb spaghetti sauce

1. Brown and crumble the ground beef in a large, heavy skillet. As the grease starts to collect in the skillet, add the onion, garlic, green pepper, and mushrooms. Continue
cooking until pepper and onion are soft.
2. Pour off the excess grease. Stir in the spaghetti sauce, and serve.

Yield: 5 servings, with (if you use the lowest-carbohydrate
spaghetti sauce) 11 grams
of carbohydrates and 4.6 grams of fiber, for a total of 6.4
grams of usable carbs and
25 grams of protein.

~ This is a good supper for the family, because, again, it's
easy to add carbs
for those who want them-you eat your very meaty meat
sauce with a
good sprinkling of Parmesan, and you let the carb-eaters
have theirs over
spaghetti. Serve a big salad with it, and there's dinner.

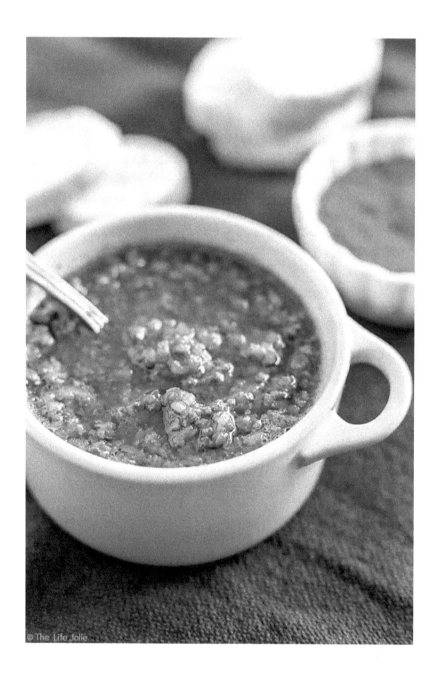

Skillet Stroganoff

1 pound ground beef
1 medium onion, diced
1 clove garlic, crushed
1 can (4 ounces) mushrooms, drained
1 teaspoon liquid beef broth concentrate
2 tablespoons Worcestershire sauce
1 teaspoon paprika
3/4 cup sour cream
Salt or Vege-Sal and pepper to taste

1. Brown and crumble the ground beef in a heavy skillet over medium heat. Add the onion and garlic as soon as there's a little grease in the bottom of the pan, and cook until all pinkness is gone from the ground beef.
2. Drain the excess grease. Add the mushrooms, broth concentrate, Worcestershire, and paprika. Stir in the sour cream, then add salt and pepper to taste. Heat through, but don't let it boil. This is great as-is, but you may certainly serve it over noodles for the non-low-carb set.

Yield: 3 servings, each with 9 grams of carbohydrates and 2 grams of fiber, for a
total of 7 grams of usable carbs and 28 grams of protein.

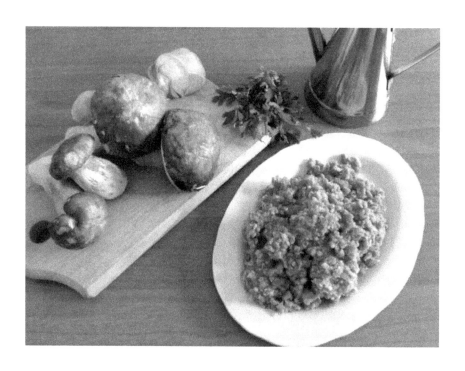

Ground Beef Helper

When your family starts agitating for the "normal" food of yore, whip up this recipe.

1 pound lean ground beef or ground turkey
1/2 cup chopped green pepper
1/2 cup chopped onion
1/2 cup diced celery
2 cans (8 ounces each) tomato sauce
2 cloves garlic, crushed; 1 teaspoon minced garlic;
or 1/2 teaspoon garlic powder
1/2 teaspoon Italian seasoning
2 cups shredded Cheddar or Monterey Jack cheese
1 box (about 1 3/4 ounces) low-carb pasta
1/3 cup water
Salt and pepper to taste

1. In a large, oven-safe skillet, brown the meat with the pepper, onion, and celery. Drain off the grease.
2. Add the tomato sauce, garlic, seasoning, 1 cup of the cheese, pasta, water, and salt and pepper to taste. Cover and simmer over low heat for 10 minutes. Turn on broiler to preheat during last the few minutes of cooking time.
3. Stir well. Spread the remaining 1 cup of cheese over the top, and broil until the cheese starts to brown.

Yield: 6 servings, each with 11 grams of carbohydrates and 2 grams of fiber, for a
total of 9 grams of usable carbs and 36 grams of protein.

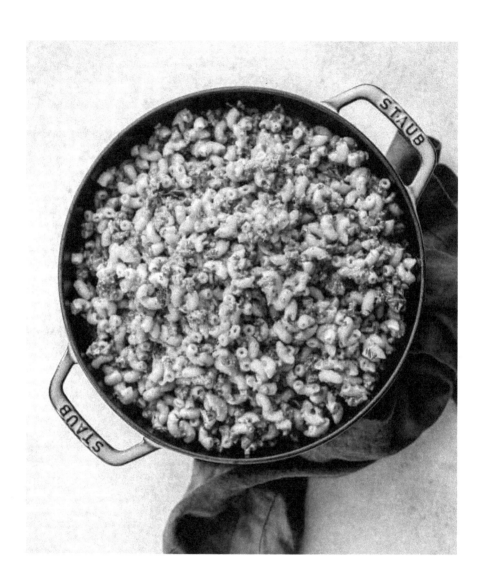

Mexican Meatballs

Marilee Wellersdick sends this easy, South-of-the-Border skillet meal.

1 pound ground beef or ground turkey
2 eggs
1 medium onion, finely chopped
3 cloves garlic, minced
2 teaspoons ground coriander
1/2 teaspoon salt
2 tablespoons oil
1 can (14 1/2 ounces) cut or crushed tomatoes
1 can (8 ounces) tomato sauce
1 tablespoon chili powder
1/2 teaspoon ground cumin

1. Mix together the ground beef, eggs, half of the onion, two-thirds of the garlic, coriander, and salt. Shape the mixture into 2-inch balls.
2. Heat the oil in a large skillet. Add the meatballs and brown them. Add the tomatoes, tomato sauce, the remaining half of the onion, the remaining third of the garlic, chili powder, and cumin to the skillet. Cover and simmer over medium-low heat for 45 minutes.

Yield: 4 servings, each with 15 grams of carbohydrates and 3 grams of fiber, for a
total of 12 grams of usable carbs and 24 grams of protein.

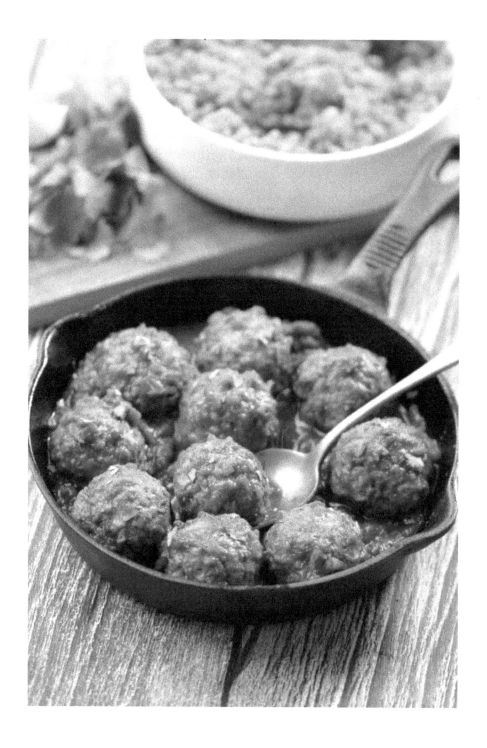

Ground Beef Stir-Fry

This looks like a lot of instructions, but it actually goes together rather quickly. It's good when you're missing Chinese food, which is generally full of added sugar and starch.

2 tablespoons soy sauce
3 tablespoons dry sherry
1 or 2 cloves garlic, crushed
1 pou nd grou nd beef
Peanut oil or other bland oil for stir-frying
1/2 cup coarsely chopped walnuts
2 cups frozen crosscut green beans, thawed, or 2 cups frozen broccoli
"cuts," thawed
1 medium onion, sliced
1 1/2 teaspoons grated fresh ginger

1. In a bowl, combine 1 tablespoon soy sauce, 4 1/2 teaspoons sherry, and the garlic. Add the ground beef and, with clean hands, mix the flavorings into the meat.

~ Remember the Law of Stir-Frying: Have everything chopped, thawed, sliced, and prepped before you start cooking!

2. Heat 2 to 3 tablespoons oil in a wok or large, heavy skillet over high heat. Put the walnuts in the skillet and fry for a few minutes, until crispy. Drain and put aside.
3. Using the same oil, stir-fry bite-size chunks of the ground beef mixture until done through. Lift out the beef, and drain.
4. Pour the oil and fat out of the skillet, and put a few tablespoons of fresh oil in. Heat it up over high heat, and add the green beans, onion, and ginger. Stir-fry until the vegetables are tender-crisp.
5. Add the beef back to the pan, and stir everything up. Stir in the remaining soy sauce and sherry, and another clove of crushed garlic if you like.

---

6. Serve without rice for you and on top of rice for the carb-eaters in the family. Sprinkle the toasted walnuts on top of each serving, and pass the soy sauce at the table for those who like more.

Yield: 3 servings, each with 19 grams of carbohydrates and 6 grams of fiber, for a
total of 13 grams of usable carbs and 34 grams of protein.

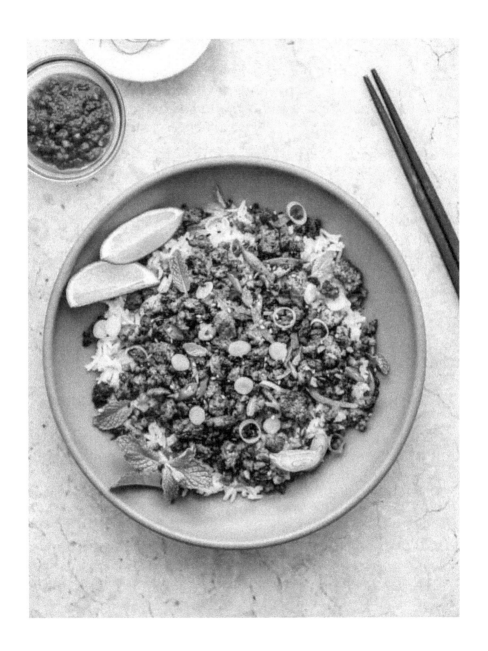

Burger Scramble Florentine

The only name I have to attribute this to is "Dottie," which is too bad, because my sister, who tested this recipe, says it's great.

1 1/2 pounds lean ground beef
1/2 cup onion, finely diced
10 ounces frozen spinach, thawed and drained
1 package (8 ounces) cream cheese, softened
1/2 cup heavy cream
1/2 cup shredded Parmesan cheese
Salt and pepper

1. Preheat the oven to 350°F. Spray a large casserole with nonstick cooking spray.
2. In a large skillet, brown the ground beef and onion. Add the spinach and cook until the meat is done.
3. In a bowl, combine the cream cheese, heavy cream, Parmesan , and salt and pepper to taste. Mix well.
4. Combine the cream cheese mixture and the meat mixture, and spoon into the prepared casserole. Bake, uncovered, for 30 minutes or until bubbly and browned on top.

Yield: 6 servings, each with 5 grams of carbohydrates and 2 grams of fiber, for a
total of 3 grams of usable carbs and 28 grams of protein.
Garden Burger Scramble. Substitute a 10-ounce package of frozen green beans
for the spinach, and use Garden Vegetable Cream Cheese instead of plain.

Yield: 6 servings, each with 6 grams of carbohydrates and 2 grams of fiber, for a
total of 4 grams of usable carbs and 28 grams of protein .

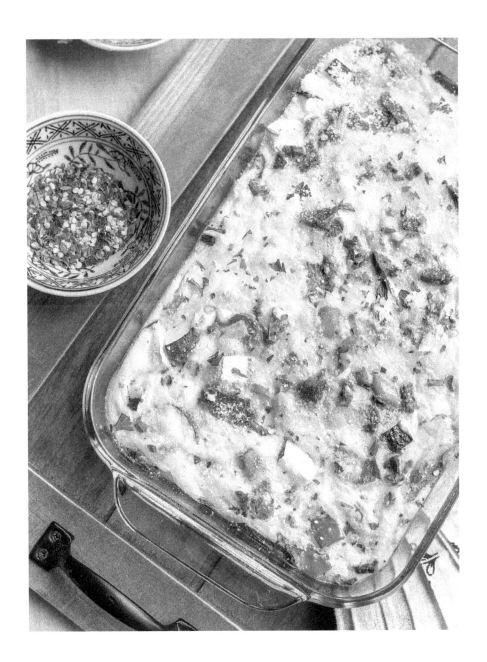

Green Bean Spaghetti

This recipe comes from Lowcarbezine! reader Marcia McCance, and it's a great dish if you're craving Italian food. If you use French cut green beans, they'll remind you more of spaghetti.

1 package (12 ounces) frozen green beans
2 to 3 tablespoons olive oil
1 small onion, chopped
1 green pepper, diced
4 or 5 medium mushrooms, sliced
1 pound ground beef, turkey, or chicken
Salt
1 can (4 ounces) plain tomato sauce
1 tablespoon Italian seasoning
Parmesan cheese

1. Cook the green beans according to package directions.
2. While the beans are cooking, put the olive oil in a large, heavy skillet over medium heat and saute the onion, green pepper, and mushrooms until the onion is translucent.
3. Add the ground beef, cook, and stir, crumbling the meat until all pinkness is gone. Sa It to taste.
4. Add the tomato sauce and the Italian seasoning. Bring to a boil, reduce to a simmer, and cook for about 5 minutes. Do not overcook.
5. Drain your green beans, pour the meat sauce over them, top with Parmesan, and serve.

Yield: 4 servings, each with 19 grams of carbohydrates and 5 grams of fiber, for a
total of 14 grams of usable carbs and 26 grams of protein.

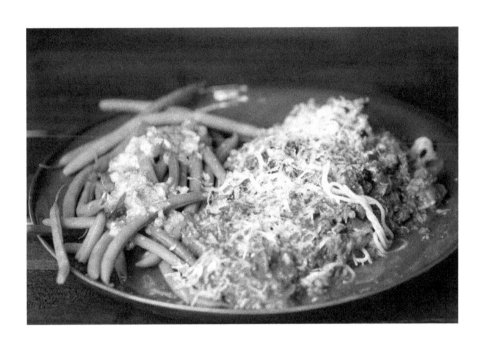

Meatza!

Here's a dish for all you pizza-lovers, and I know you are legion. Just add a salad, and you have a supper that will please the whole family.

1 1/2 pounds ground beef or 3/4 pound ground beef mixed with 3/4 pound
Italian-style sausage
1 small onion, finely chopped
1 clove garlic, crushed
1 teaspoon dried oregano or Italian seasoning (optional)
8 ounces sugar-free pizza sauce
Parmesan or Romano cheese (optional)
8 ounces shredded mozzarella
Toppings (peppers, onions, mushrooms, or whatever you like)
Olive oil (optional)

1. Preheat the oven to 350°F.
2. In a large bowl and with clean hands, combine the meat with the onion and garlic, and a teaspoon of oregano or Italian seasoning (if using). Mix well.
3. Pat the meat mixture out in an even layer in a 9 x 12-inch baking pan. Bake for 20 minutes.
4. When the meat comes out, it will have shrunk a fair amount, because of the grease cooking off. Pour off the grease and spread the pizza sauce over the meat. Sprinkle the Parmesan on the sauce (if using), and then distribute the shredded mozzarella evenly over the sauce.
5. Top with whatever you like: green peppers, banana peppers, mushrooms, olives, anchovies. I love broccoli on pizza, and thawed frozen broccoli "cuts" work perfectly. You could also use meat toppings, such as sausage and pepperoni, but they seem a little redundant, since the whole bottom layer is meat.
6. Drizzle the whole thing with a little olive oil (if using; it's really not necessary).

7. Put your Meatza! 4 inches below a broiler set on High. Broil for about 5 minutes, or until the cheese is melted and starting to brown.

*Yield: 6 servings, each with about 5 grams of carbohydrates
per serving, only a trace
of fiber, and 27 grams of protein. (Based on using sugar-free pizza sauce, and only
cheese, no veggies.)*

*~ If you haven't been able to find a pizza sauce that doesn't have sugar,
you might combine an 8-ounce can of tomato sauce with a crushed clove
of garlic and some oregano.*

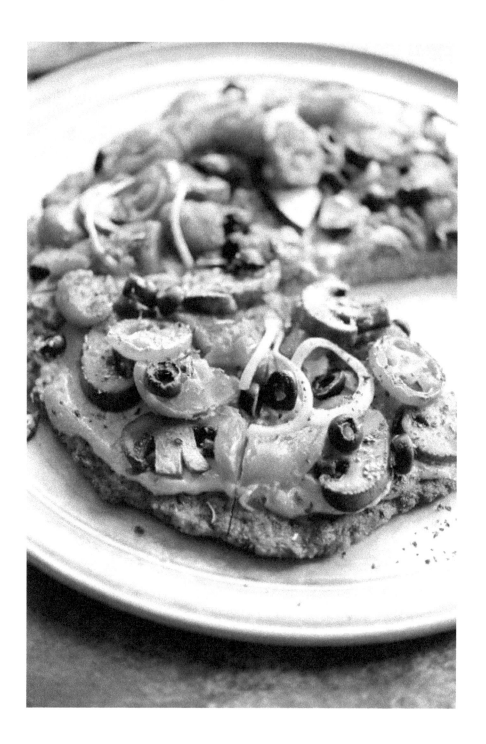

Joe

Our favorite one-dish skillet supper. It's flexible, too; don't worry if you use a little less or a little more burger, or one more or one fewer egg.
It'll still come out great.

1 1/2 pounds ground beef
1 package (10 ounces) frozen chopped spinach
1 medium onion, chopped
1 or 2 cloves garlic, crushed
5 eggs
Salt and pepper

1. In a heavy skillet over a medium flame, begin browning the ground beef.
2. While the beef is cooking, cook the spinach according to the package directions (or 5 to 7 minutes on high in the microwave should do it).
3. When the ground beef is half done, add the onion and garlic, and cook until the beef is completely done. Pour off the extra fat.
4. Drain the sp inach well-I put mine in a strainer and press it with the back of a spoon-and stir it into the ground beef.
5. Mix up the eggs well with a fork, and stir them in with the beef and spinach. Continue cooking and stirring over low heat for a few more minutes, until the eggs are set. Salt and pepper to taste, and serve.

Yield: 6 servings, each with 4 grams of carbohydrates and 2 grams of fiber, for a
total of 2 grams of usable carbs and 25 grams of protein.

~ My sister likes a little Parmesan cheese sprinkled over her Joe, and I surely
wouldn't argue about a little thing like that!

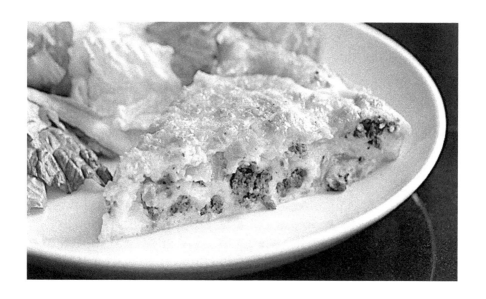

Sloppy Jose

So easy it's almost embarrassing, and the kids will probably like it. Different brands of Salsa vary a lot in their carb contents, so read labels carefully.

1 pound ground beef
1 cup salsa (mild, medium, or hot, as you prefer)
1 cup shredded Mexican-style cheese

1. In a large skillet, crumble and brown the ground beef, and drain off the fat.
2. Stir in the salsa and cheese, and heat until the cheese is melted.

Yield: About 4 servings, each with 4 grams of carbohydrates and 1 gram of fiber, for
a total of 3 grams of usable carbs and 27 grams of protein.
Mega Sloppy Jose. Try adding another 1/2 cup salsa and another 1/2 cup cheese.

Yield: 4 servings, each with 6 grams of carbohydrates and 2 grams of fiber, for a
total of 4 grams of usable carbs and 30 grams of protein.

This is good with a salad, or even on a salad. Of course, if you have carbeaters
around, they'll love the stuff on some corn tortillas.

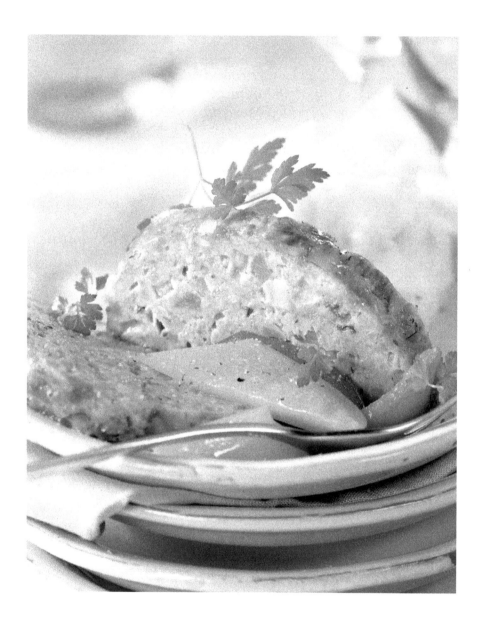

All-Meat Chili

Some folks consider tomatoes in chili to be anathema, but I like it this way. Don't look funny at that cocoa powder, by the way. It's the secret ingredient!

2 pou nds grou nd beef
1 cup chopped onion
3 cloves garlic, crushed
1 can (14 1/2 ounces) tomatoes with green chilies
1 can (4 ounces) plain tomato sauce
4 teaspoons ground cumin
2 teaspoons dried oregano
2 teaspoons unsweetened cocoa powder
1 teaspoon paprika

1. Brown and crumble the beef in a heavy skillet over medium-high heat. Pour off the grease, and add the onion, garlic, tomatoes, tomato sauce, cumin , oregano, cocoa, and paprika. Stir to combine.
2. Turn the burner to low, cover, and simmer for 30 minutes. Uncover and simmer for another 15 to 20 minutes, or until the chili thickens a bit. Serve with grated cheese, sour cream, chopped raw onion, or other low-carb toppings.

Yield: 6 servings, each with 7 grams of carbohydrates and 2 grams of fiber, for a
total of 5 grams of usable carbs and 27 grams of protein.

It's easy to vary this recipe to the tastes of different family members. If
some people like beans in their chili, just heat up a can of kidney or pinto
beans, and let them spoon their beans into their own serving. If you like
beans in your chili, buy a can of black soybeans at a health food store;
there are only a couple of grams of usable carbs in a couple of tablespoons.

And of course, if you like your chili hotter than this, just add crushed red
pepper, cayenne, or hot sauce to take things up a notch.

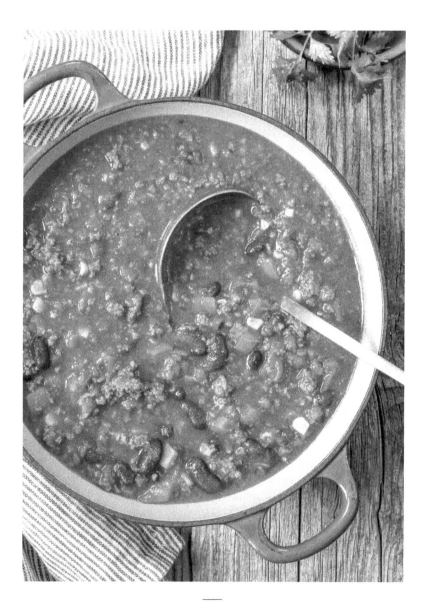

Mexicali Meat Loaf

1 pound ground beef
1 pound mild pork sausage
1 cup crushed plain pork rinds
1 can (4 1/2 ounces) diced mild green chilies
1 medium onion, finely chopped
8 ounces Monterey Jack cheese, cut into 1/4- to 1/2-inch
cubes or shredded
3/4 cup salsa (mild, medium, or hot, as desired)
1 egg
2 or 3 cloves garlic, crushed
2 teaspoons dried oregano
2 teaspoons ground cumin
1 teaspoon salt or Vege-Sal
1. Preheat the oven to 350°F.

1. Combine all these ingredients in a really big bowl, and then, with clean hands, knead it all until it's thoroughly blended .
2. Dump it out on a clean broiler rack, and form into a loaf-it'll be a big loaf-about
3 inches thick. Bake for 1 1/2 hours.

~ Do chop the onion quite fine for your meat loaves. If it's in pieces that are
too big, it tends to make the loaf fall apart when you cut it.
The Mexicali
Meat Loaf may crumble a bit anyway, because it's quite tender.

Yield: 8 servings, each with 5 grams of carbohydrates and 1 gram of fiber, for a total
of 4 grams of usable carbs and 28 grams of protein.

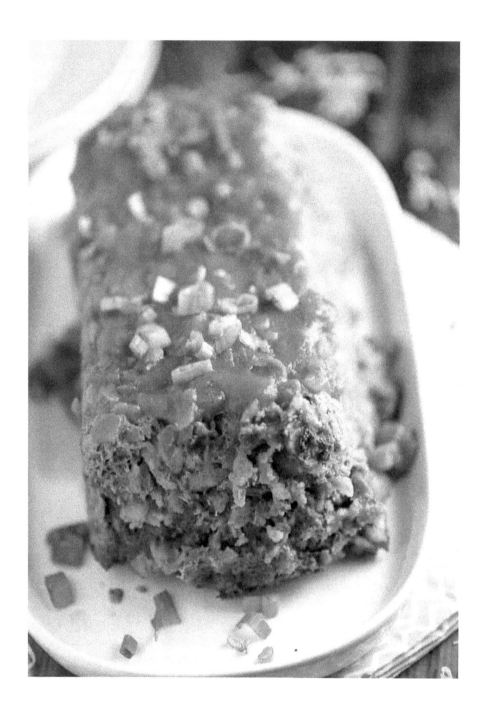

Low-Carb Swiss Loaf

I adapted this from a recipe that had a whole pile of bread crumbs and a cup of milk in it. I simply left them out, and I've never missed them.

2 1/2 pounds ground beef
5 ounces Swiss cheese, diced small or grated
2 eggs, beaten
1 medium onion, chopped
1 green pepper, chopped
1 small rib celery, chopped
1 teaspoon salt or Vege-Sal
1/2 teaspoon pepper
1/2 teaspoon paprika

1. Preheat the oven to 350°F.
2. With clean hands, combine all the ingredients in a large bowl, until the mixture is well blended.
3. Pack the meat into one large loaf pan or two small ones. Bake a large loaf for 1 ½ to 1 3/4 hours. Bake two small loaves for 1 1/4 hours.

~ I turn the loaf out of the pan and onto the broiler rack, and I bake it there
so the excess fat runs off-not because I'm afraid of fat, but because I like
it better that way. If you like, though, you could bake yours right in the
pan, and it would probably be a bit more tender.

Yield: 8 servings, each with 3 grams of carbohydrates and 1 gram of fiber, for a total
of 2 grams of usable carbs and 30 grams of protein.

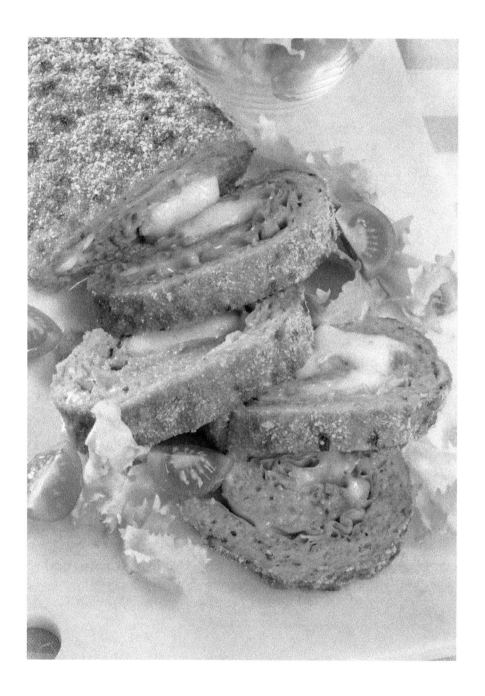

46

Zucchini Meat Loaf Italiano

The inspiration for this meat loaf was a recipe in an Italian cookbook. The original recipe was for a "zucchini mold," and it had only a tiny bit of meat in it. I thought to myself, "How could adding more ground beef be a problem here?" And I was right; it's very moist and flavorful.

3 tablespoons olive oil
2 medium zucchini, chopped (about 1 1/2 cups)
1 medium onion, chopped
2 or 3 cloves garlic, crushed
1 1/2 pounds ground beef
2 tablespoons snipped fresh parsley
1 egg
3/4 cup grated Parmesan cheese
1 teaspoon salt
1/2 teaspoon pepper

1. Preheat the oven to 350°F.
2. Heat the olive oil in a skillet and saute the zucchini, onion, and garlic in it for 7 to 8 mi nutes.
3. Let the veggies cool a bit, then put them in a big bowl with the beef, parsley, egg, cheese, salt, and pepper. Using clean hands, mix thoroughly.
4. Take the rather soft meat mixture and put it in a big loaf pan, if you like, or form the loaf right on a broiler rack so the grease will drip off. (Keep in mind if you do it this way, your loaf won't stand very high, it'll be about 2 inches thick.)
5. Bake for 75 to 90 minutes, or until the juices run clear but the loaf is not dried out.

Yield: 5 servings, each with 3 grams of carbohydrates and 1 gram of fiber, for total of 2 grams of usable carbs and 29 grams of protein.

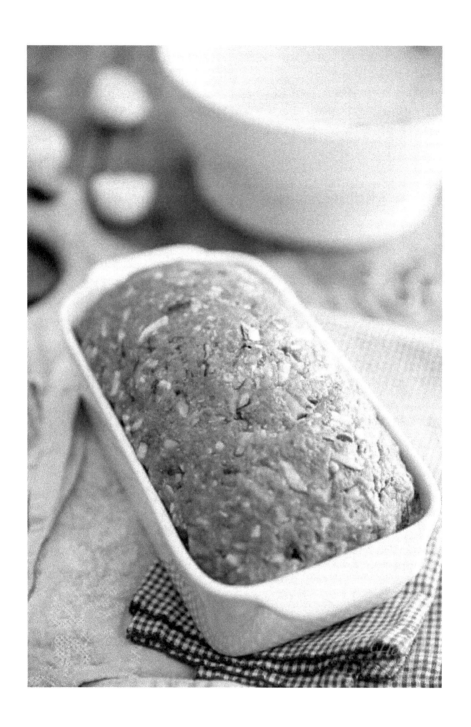

My Grandma's Standby Casserole

Okay, my grandma used egg noodles instead of spaghetti squash, but it tastes good this way, too. This is handy for potlucks and such.

1 pou nd grou nd beef
2 tablespoons butter
1 clove garlic, crushed
1 teaspoon salt
Dash pepper
2 cans (8 ounces each) plain tomato sauce
6 scallions
3 ounces cream cheese
1 cup sour cream
3 cups cooked spaghetti squash
1/2 cup shredded Cheddar cheese

1. Preheat the oven to 350°F.
2. Brown the ground beef in the butter. Pour off the grease, and stir in the garlic, salt, pepper, and tomato sauce.
3. Cover, turn the burner to low, and simmer for 20 minutes.
4. While the meat is simmering, slice the scallions, including the crisp part of the green, and combine with the cream cheese and sour cream. Blend well.
5. In the bottom of a 6-cup casserole, layer half the spaghetti squash, half the scallion mixture, and half the tomato-beef mixture; repeat the layers. Top with the Cheddar, and bake for 20 minutes.

Yield: 5 servings, each with 15 grams of carbohydrates and 2 grams of fiber, for a
total of 13 grams of usable carbs and 23 grams of protein.

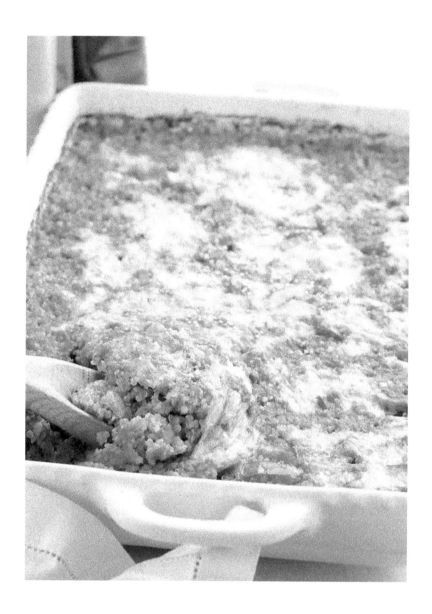

BeefTaco Filling

1 pound ground beef
2 tablespoons Taco Seasoning
1/4 cup water

1. Brown and crumble the ground beef in a heavy skillet over medium-high heat.
2. When the meat is cooked through, drain the grease and stir in the seasoning and water. Let it simmer for about 5 minutes, and serve.

Yield: 4 servings, each with less than 1 gram of carbohydrates, no fiber, and 19 grams of protein.

Use in the Taco Omelets Taco Salads, Cheesy Bowls and Taco Shells and Tortillas

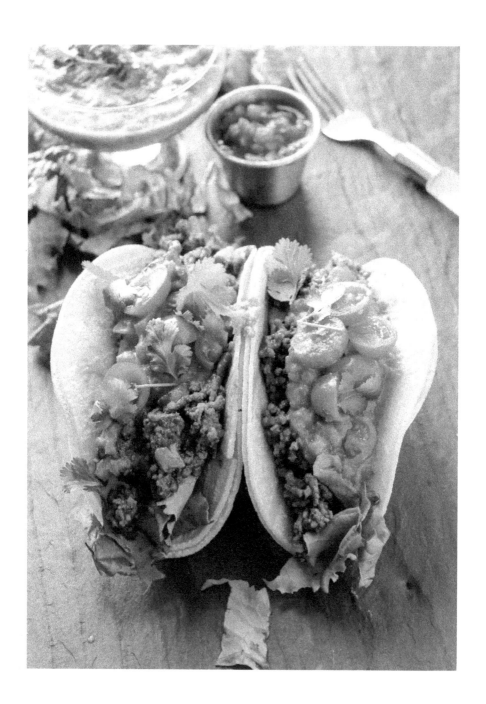

Reuben Casserole

Another great recipe from Vicki Cash. Thanks, Vicki!

4 small summer squash or zucchini
2 tablespoons water
1 can (27 ounces) sauerkraut, drained
1 tablespoon caraway seeds
2 tablespoons Dijon mustard
8 ounces shaved corned beef or pastrami
4 ounces grated Swiss cheese

1. Slice the squash into bite-size pieces. Place the pieces in a 2-quart microwave-safe casserole, and add the water. Cover and microwave on High for 3 minutes.

2. Add the sauerkraut, caraway seeds, mustard, and meat, mixing well. Cover and microwave on High for 6 minutes, stirring halfway through.

3. Stir in the cheese, and microwave for 3 to 5 more minutes, or until the cheese is melted.

Yield: 4 servings, each with 16 grams of carbohydrates and 8 grams of fiber, for a
total of 8 grams of usable carbs and 21 grams of protein.

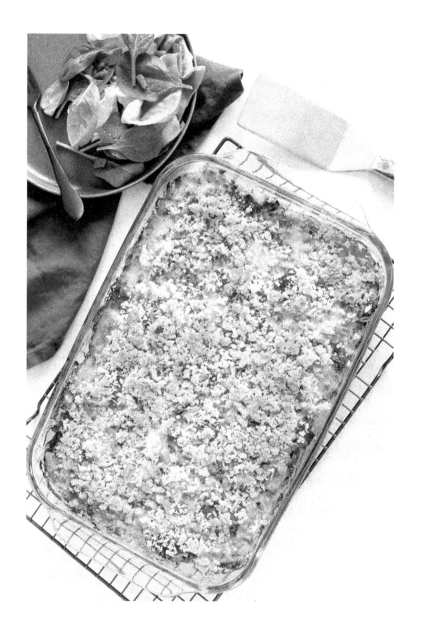

Beef Fajitas

This is my take on a recipe sent to me by Carol Vandiver. You can serve these with low-carb tortillas, if you like, but I just pile mine on a plate, top them with salsa, sour cream, and guac, and eat 'em with a fork.

1/2 cup lite beer
1/2 cup oil
2 tablespoons lime juice
1/2 small onion, thinly sliced
1 teaspoon red pepper flakes
1/4 teaspoon ground cumin
1/4 teaspoon pepper
1 1/2 pounds skirt steak
1 tablespoon oil
1 medium onion, thickly sliced
1 green pepper, cut into strips
Low-carb tortillas, purchased, or homemade
Guacamole
Salsa
Sour cream

1. Mix together the beer, oil, lime juice, onion, pepper flakes, cumin, and pepper; this is your marinade.
2. Place the skirt steak in a large zipper-lock bag, and pour the marinade over it. Seal the bag, pressing out the air, and put it in the fridge. Let your steak marinate for a minimum of several hours.
3. When you're ready to cook, remove your steak from the bag, reserving a couple of tablespoons of the marinade. Slice your steak quite thin, across the grain.
4. Add the oil to a large, heavy skillet over high heat, and tilt to coat the bottom. When. the skillet is good and hot, add the steak slices, onion, and pepper. Stir-fry them until the meat is done through and the vegetables are crisp-tender. S. Stir in the reserved marinade, and serve, with or without low-carb tortillas, topped with guacamole, salsa, and sour cream.

Yield: 4 servings, each with about 5 grams of carbohydrates and 1 gram of fiber,
for a total of 4 grams of usable carbs and 34 grams of protein. (Analysis does not
include guacamole, sour cream, salsa, or low-carb tortillas).

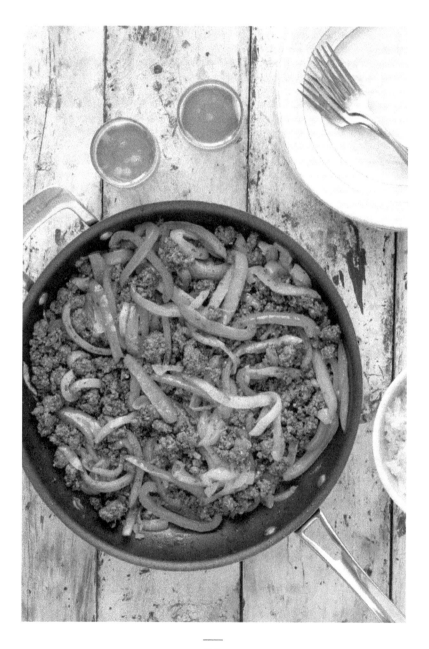

Steakhouse Steak

Ever wonder why steak is better at a steakhouse than it is at home? Part of it is that the best grades of meat are reserved for the restaurants, but it's also the method: quick grilling, at very high heat, very close to the flame. Try it at home, with this recipe.

Olive oil
1 1/2 to 2 pounds well-marbled steak (sirloin, rib eye, or the like),
1 to 1 1/2 inches thick

1. Rub a couple of teaspoons of olive oil on either side of the steak.
2. Arrange your broiler so you can get the steak so close that it's almost, but not quite, touching the broiling element. (I have to put my broiler pan on top of a skillet turned upside down to do this.) Turn the broiler to high, and get that steak in there. Leave the oven door open-this is crucial. For a 1-inch thick steak, set the oven timer for 5 to 5 1/2 minutes; for a 1 1/2-inch-thick steak, you can go up to 6 minutes.
3. When the timer beeps, quickly flip the steak, and set the timer again. Check at this point to see if your time seems right. If you like your steak a lot rarer or more welldone than I do, or if you have a different brand of broiler, you may need to adjust how long you broil the second side for.
4. When the timer goes off again, get that steak out of there quickly, put it on a serving plate, and season it any way you like.

Yield: The number of servings will depend on the size of your steak, but what you
really need to know is that there are no carbs here at all.

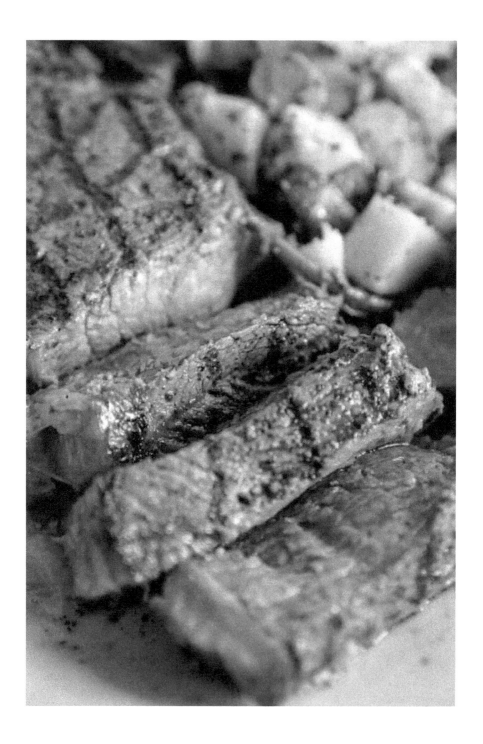

Southwestern Steak

I adore steak, I adore guacamole, and the combination is fantastic.

Olive oil
1 1/2 to 2 pounds well -marbled steak (sirloin, rib eye, or the like),
1 to 1 1/2 inches thick
Guacamole
Salt and pepper

Prepare the Steakhouse Steak to your preferred degree of doneness. Spread each serving of steak with a heaping tablespoon of guacamole, and salt and pepper to taste.

Yield: The number of servings will depend on the size of your steak, but the
guacamole will add 4 grams of carbohydrates and 1 gram of fiber, for a total of
3 grams of usable carbs. You'll also get 275 milligrams of potassium.

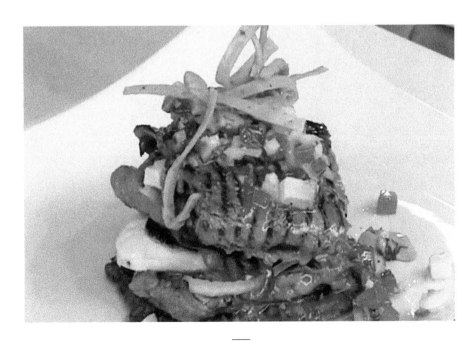

Cajun Steak

2 to 3 teaspoons Cajun Seasoning
1 pound sirloin steak, 1 inch thick

Simply sprinkle Cajun seasoning over both sides of your steak.
Then either pan-broil it (cook in on a very hot, ungreased, heavy
skillet) or cook it on a stove top grill over maximum heat. Either
way, cook it just 6 1/2 minutes per side.

Yield: 3 or 4 servings; the Cajun seasoning adds a bare trace
of carbohydrates to
each.

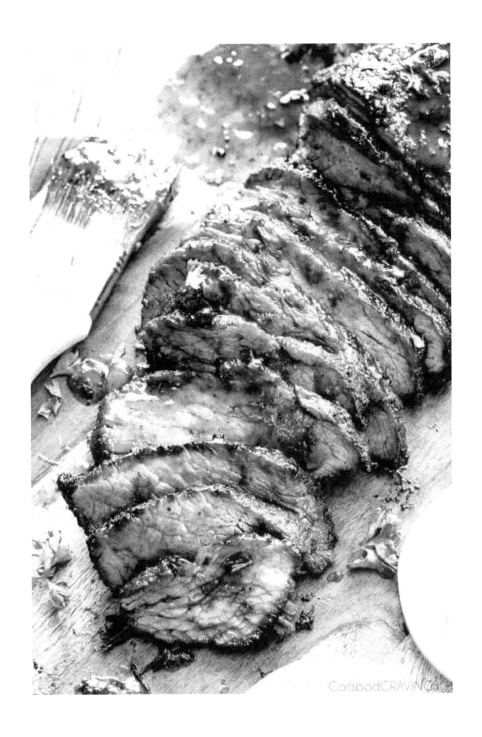

Steak Vinaigrette

You don't have to make a batch of homemade vinaigrette every time you want a steak; store-bought will work just as well here.

Steak, in your preferred cut and quantity
1/2 cup vinaigrette dressing for each pound of steak

1. Put your steak in a 1-quart zipper-lock bag, and pour the vinaigrette dressing over it. Let the steak marinate for at least 15 minutes, or leave it all day, if you have the time.
2. When you're ready to cook your steak, remove it from the bag, discard the marinade, and broil or grill it, as you prefer

Yield: Assume 1 pound of steak is 2 servings, each with about 1 gram of
carbohydrates, maximum, no fiber, and 33 grams of protein.

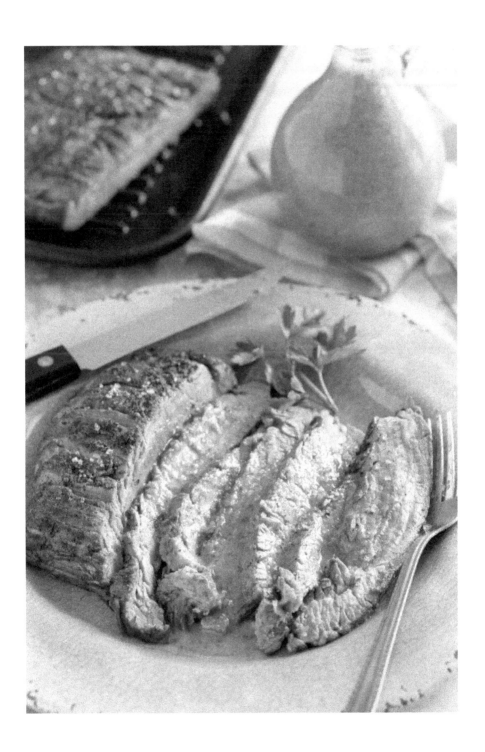

Blue Cheese Steak Butter

This is one of those recipes that would have horrified me back in my low-fat days-and it's so good! If you don't have a food processor, you can make this by hand; it will just take some vigorous mixing.

1/2 pound blue cheese, crum

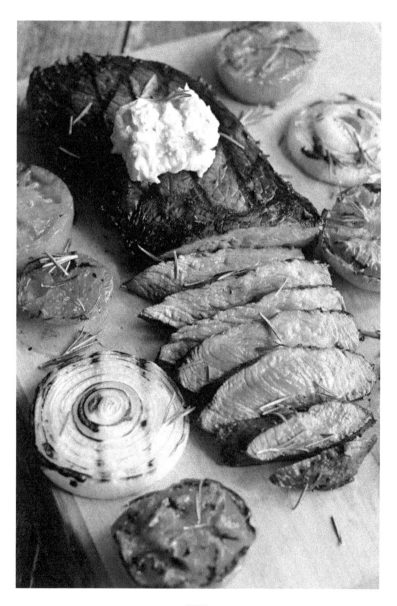

Side Dish Salad

I'm hard-pressed to think of a food that is more ill-done-by than salad. Way too many people dump some "iceberg mix" in a bowl, throw in some pink, mealy winter tomatoes, slosh some gooey bottled dressing on top, and then wail that their families show no enthusiasm for salad.

Made with just a little attention, salad is one of the most delicious, exciting foods imaginable. It is, of course, one of the most nutritious, as well, so learn to pay attention to your salads.

First of all, ditch the iceberg lettuce; not only is it the least-nutritious lettuce on the market, it's also the blandest. Try all sorts of other green and leafy things, such as romaine, Boston lettuce, butterhead, radicchio, frizzee, fresh spinach, or whatever else you can find. Try making some fresh dressings, too.

And unless all the members of your family have violently opposing opinions on salad dressing, try actually tossing your salad with the dressing, instead of just sloshing it on top. I think you'll be surprised at the difference it makes in the end product.

The dressings, by the way, are at the end of this chapter. But let's get to the salads themselves right now.

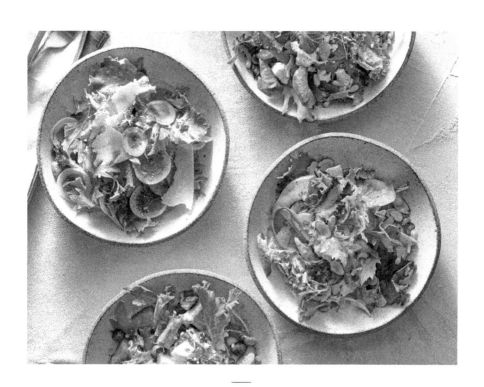

Greek Salad

This is a wonderful, filling, fresh-tasting salad we never get tired of.

1 large head romaine lettuce
1 cup chopped fresh parsley
1/2 cucumber, sliced
1 green pepper, sliced
Greek Lemon Dressing
1/4 sweet red onion, thinly sliced into rings
12 to 15 Greek olives
2 ripe tomatoes, cut into wedges
4 to 6 ounces feta cheese, crumbled
Anchovy fillets packed in olive oil (if desired)

1. Wash and dry your romaine, and break or cut it into bite-size pieces. Cut up and add the parsley, cucumber, and green pepper.

~ You can do step 1 ahead of time, if you like, which makes this salad very
doable on a weeknight.

2. Just before serving, pour on the Greek dressing, and toss the salad like crazy.
3. Arrange the onions, olives, and tomatoes artistically on top, and sprinkle the crumbled feta in the middle. You can also add the anchovies at this point, if you know that everybody likes them, but I prefer to make them available for those who like them to put on their individual serving.

Yield: 4 servings, each with 16 grams of carbohydrates and 6 grams of fiber, for a
total of 10 grams of usable carbs and 11 grams of protein.

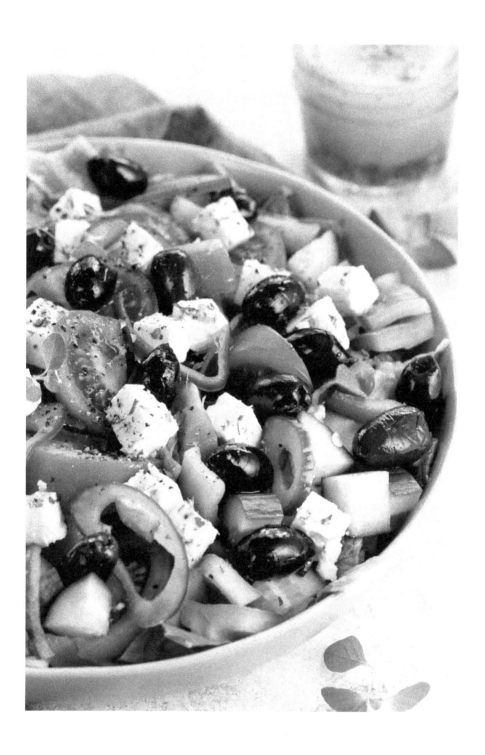

Autumn Salad

The flavor contrasts in this salad are lovely, and I've kept the pear to a quantity that won't add too many carbs.

2 tablespoons butter
1/2 cup chopped walnuts
10 cups loosely packed assorted greens (romaine, red leaf lettuce,
and fresh spinach)
1/4 sweet red onion, thinly sliced
1/4 cup olive oil
2 teaspoons wine vinegar
2 teaspoons lemon juice
1/4 teaspoon spicy brown or Dijon mustard
1/8 teaspoon salt
1/8 teaspoon pepper
1/2 ripe pear, chopped
1/3 cup crumbled blue cheese

1. Melt the butter in a small, heavy skillet over medium heat. Add the walnuts, and let them toast in the butter, stirring occasionally, for about 5 minutes.
2. While the walnuts are toasting-and make sure you keep an eye on them and don't burn them-wash and dry your greens, and put them in salad bowl with the onion.
Toss with the oil first, then combine the vinegar, lemon juice, mustard, salt, and pepper, and add that to the salad bowl. Toss until everything is well covered.
3. Top the salad with the pear, the warm toasted walnuts, and the crumbled blue cheese; serve.

*Yield: 4 generous servings, each with 13 grams of carbohydrates and 6 grams of fiber,
for a total of 7 grams of usable carbs and 10 grams of protein.*

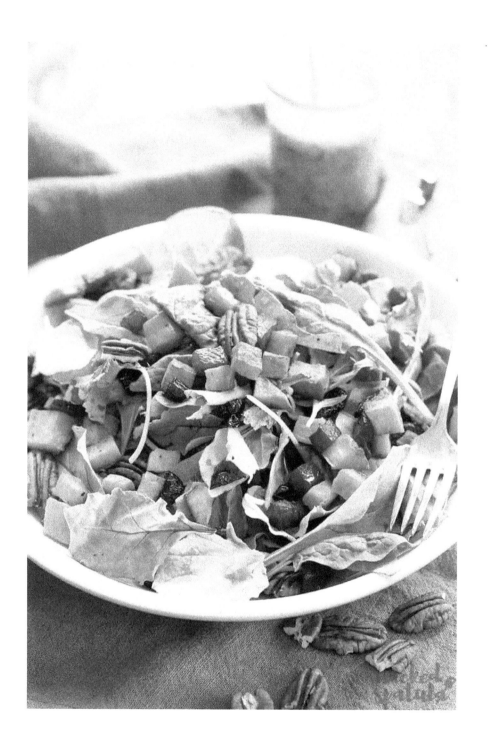

Arugula-Pear Salad

An extraordinary combination of flavors. If you've never tried arugula, you'll be surprised: It tastes almost as if it's been roasted. You could use grated Parmesan cheese, but I think the bigger pieces of thinly sliced

Parmesan make a difference in the salad's flavor.
3 1/2 to 4 cups washed, dried, torn-up arugula
1/2 ripe pear, cut in small chunks or slices
3 tablespoons extra-virgin olive oil
Juice of 1 lemon
Salt and pepper
2 tablespoons very thinly sliced bits of Parmesan cheese

Combine the arugula and pear in a salad bowl. Add the olive oil, and toss well. Add the lemon juice, salt and pepper lightly, and toss again. Top with Parmesan, and serve.

Yield: 2 generous servings, each with 9 grams of
carbohydrates and 2 grams of fiber,
for a total of 7 grams of usable carbs and 3 grams of protein.

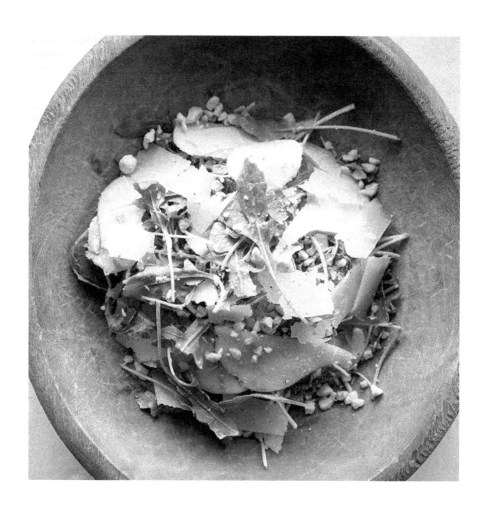

Spinach Pecan Salad

2 pounds fresh spi nach
Salt or Vege-Sal
10 scallions, thinly sliced, including about 2 inches of the
green sprout
1/4 cup extra-virgin olive oil
1/4 cup lemon juice
1/4 pound toasted, salted pecans, chopped

1. Wash and dry the spinach until you're absolutely sure it's clean-spinach can hold a lot of grit! When you're sure it's clean and dry, put it in a salad bowl, and sprinkle it with a little salt-maybe a teaspoonful-and squeeze the leaves gently with your hands. You'll find that the spinach "deflates," or sort of gets a bit limp and reduces in volume. Add the scallions to the bowl.
2. Pour on the olive oil, and toss the salad thoroughly. Add the lemon juice, and toss again. Top with the pecans, and serve.

Yield: 6 servings, each with 12 grams of carbohydrates and 6 grams of fiber, for a
total of 6 grams of usable carbs and 6 grams of protein.

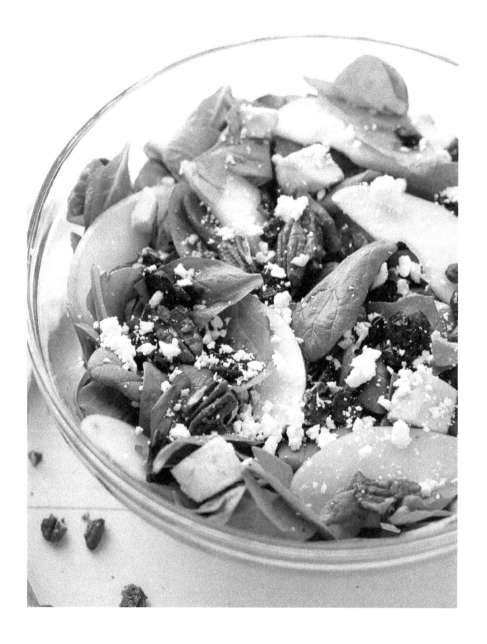

Classic Spinach Salad

4 cups fresh spinach
1/8 large, sweet red onion, thinly sliced
3 tablespoons oil
2 tablespoons apple cider vinegar
2 teaspoons tomato paste
1 1/2 teaspoons Splenda
1/4 small onion, grated
1/8 teaspoon dry mustard
Salt and pepper
2 slices bacon, cooked until crisp, and crumbled
1 hard-boiled egg, chopped

1. Wash the spinach very well, and dry. Tear up larger leaves. Combine with the onion inasalad bowl.
2. In a separate bowl, mix up the oil, vinegar, tomato paste, Splenda, onion, mustard, and salt and pepper to taste. Pour the mixture over the spinach and onion, and toss.
3. Top the salad with the bacon and egg, and serve.

*Yield: 2 generous servings, each with 7 grams of carbohydrates and 2 grams of fiber,
for a total of 5 grams of usable carbs and 2 grams of protein.*

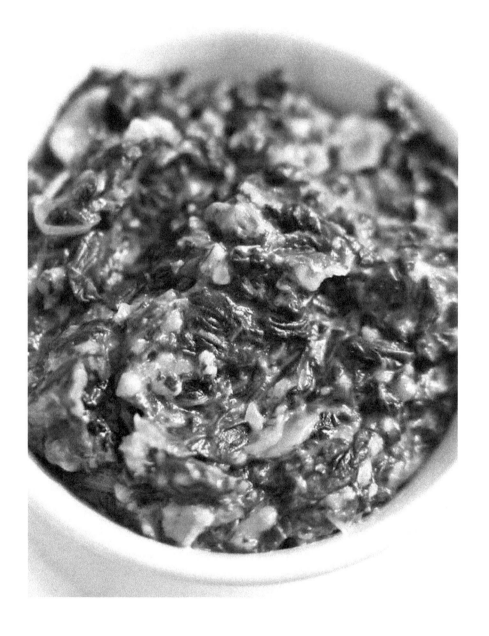

Summer Treat Spinach Salad

Worried about where you'll get your potassium now that you're not eating bananas? Each serving of this salad has more potassium than three bananas!

2 pounds raw spinach
1 ripe avocado
1/4 cantaloupe
1/2 cup alfalfa sprouts
2 scallions, sliced
French Vinaigrette Dressing

1. Wash the spinach very well, and dry. Tear up larger leaves.
2. Cut the avocado in half, remove the pit and the peel, and cut into chunks.
3. Peel and chunk the cantaloupe, or, if you want to be fancy, use a melon bailer.
4. Add the avocado and cantaloupe to the spinach, along with the alfalfa sprouts and scallions. Toss with the vinaigrette right before serving.

Yield: 6 servings, each with 11 grams of carbohydrates and 5 grams of fiber, for a
total of 6 grams of usable carbs and 5 grams of protein.

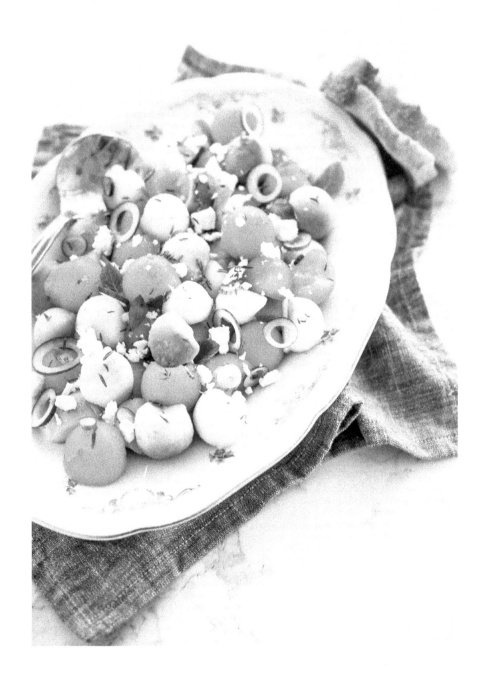

Mixed Greens with Warm Brie Dressing

This elegant dinner party fare is a carbohydrate bargain with lotsof flavor.

1 1/2 quarts torn romaine lettuce, washed and dried
1 1/2 quarts torn red leaf lettuce, washed and dried
2 cups torn radicchio, washed and dried
1 cup chopped fresh parsley
4 scallions, thinly sliced, including the crisp part of the green shoot
1/2 cup extra-virgin olive oil
1/2 small onion, minced
3 cloves garlic, crushed
6 ounces Brie, rind removed, cut into small chunks
1/4 cup sherry vinegar
1 tablespoon lemon juice
1 1/2 teaspoons Dijon mustard

1. Put the lettuce, radicchio, parsley, and scallions in a large salad bowl, and keep cold.
2. Put the olive oil in a heavy-bottomed saucepan over medium-low heat. Add the onion and garlic, and let them cook for 2 to 3 minutes.
3. Melt in the Brie, one chunk at a time, continuously stirring with a whisk. (It'll look dreadful at first, but don't sweat it.)
4. When all the cheese is melted in, whisk in the sherry vinegar, lemon juice, and
Dijon mustard. Let it cook for a few minutes, stirring all the while, until your dressing is smooth and thick. Pour over the salad and toss.

Yield: 6 servings, each with 7 grams of carbohydrates and 3 of fiber, for a total of
4 grams of usable carbs and 8 grams of protein.

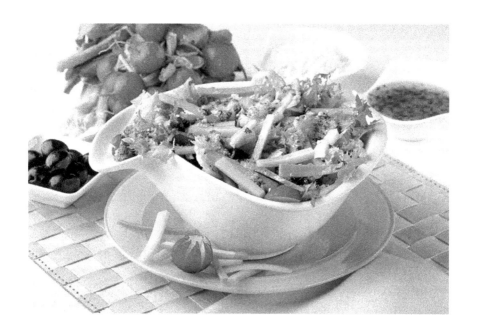

Bayside Salad

This is my version of a fantastic salad I had at a restaurant called The Bayside Grill, down near the Gulf Coast. The combination of greens isn't vital-you can change it some, as long as you make sure to include some bitter greens, such as endive.

2 tablespoons butter
1/4 cup chopped pecans
2 cups torn romaine
1 cup torn radicchio
1 cup torn frizee
1 cup torn Boston lettuce
1 cup torn curly endive
1/4 sweet red onion, thinly sliced
Raspberry Vinaigrette
1/4 cup crumbled blue cheese
4 slices bacon, cooked until crisp

1. Melt the butter in a heavy skillet. Add the pecans and toast them over medium heat, stirring for 5 minutes or so, until brown and crisp.
2. Toss the romaine, radicchio, frizee, Boston lettuce, curly endive, and onion with the Raspberry Vinaigrette.
3. Pile the salad on 4 serving plates, and top each with 1 tablespoon of pecans, 1 tablespoon of blue cheese, and 1 crumbled slice of bacon.

Yield: 4 servings, each with 6 grams of carbohydrates and 2 grams of fiber, for a
total of 4 grams of usable carbs and 2 grams of protein.

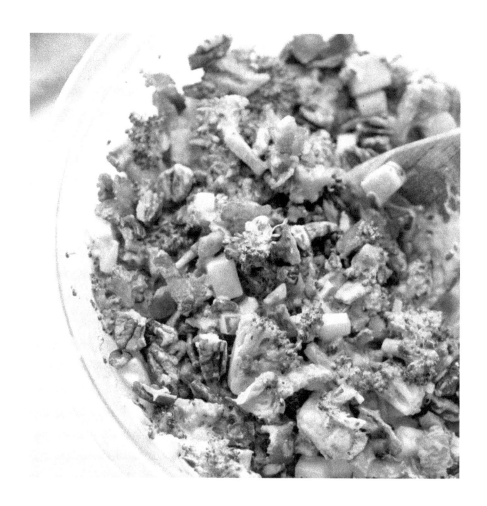

Caesar Salad

This is the salad that made Tijuana restaurateur Caesar Cardini famous. If you've only had that wilted stuff that passes for Caesar salad on salad bars and buffets, you have to try this.

1 large head romaine lettuce
Caesar Dressing

Wash, dry, and tear up an entire head of romaine lettuce. Toss it with the dressing. That's it!

Yield: 6 servings, each with 5 grams of carbohydrates and 2 grams of fiber, for a
total of 3 grams of usable carbs and 6 grams of protein.

~ If you're feeling particularly spiffy and you have some low-carb bread on hand, you could dice up a couple of slices, put them in a pan with 1/4 cup of olive oil and a couple of cloves of garlic, and saute them for a few minutes, until they're brown and crispy. But me, I'd only bother with that for company.

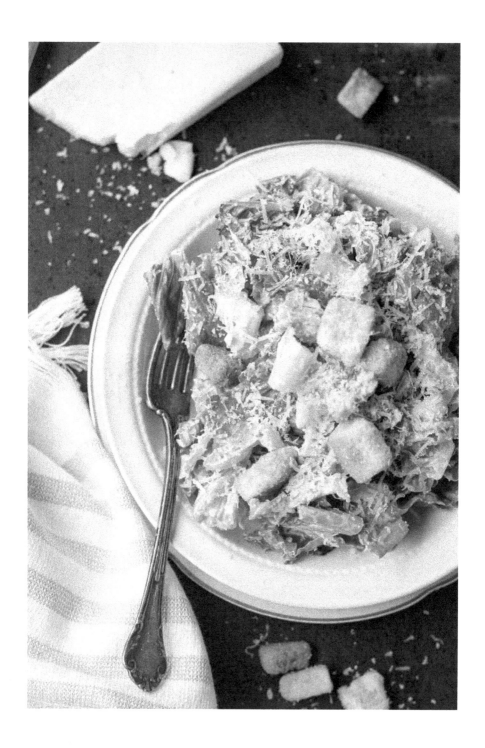

Our Favorite Salad

We've served this salad over and over, and we never tire of it. This dressing tastes a lot like Caesar, but it's less trouble, and there's no blender to wash afterwards.

1 clove garlic
1/2 cup extra-virgin olive oil
1 head romaine
1/2 cup chopped fresh parsley
1/2 green pepper, diced
1/4 cucumber, quartered and sliced
1/4 sweet red onion
2 to 3 tablespoons lemon juice
2 to 3 teaspoons Worcestershire sauce
1/4 cup Parmesan cheese
1 medium ripe tomato, cut into thin wedges

1. (rush the clove of garlic in a small bowl, cover it with the olive oil, and set it aside.
2. Wash and dry your romaine, break it up into a bowl, and add the parsley, pepper, cucumber, and onion. Pour the garlic-flavored oil over the salad, and toss until every leaf is covered.
3. Sprinkle on the lemon juice, and toss again. Then sprinkle on the Worcestershire sauce, and toss again. Finally, sprinkle on the Parmesan, and toss one last time. Top with the tomatoes, and serve.

Yield: 6 servings, each with 7 grams of carbohydrates and 3 grams of fiber, for a
total of 4 grams of usable carbs and 4 grams of protein.

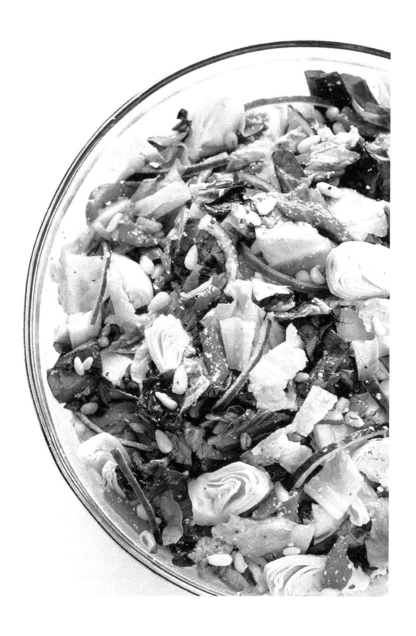

Update Salad

This recipe went around in the 1960s, using curly endive instead of this mixture of bitter greens, and of course, using sugar in the dressing.
I like to think I've brought it into the 21st century-hence the name.

Salad
2 medium green peppers, cut in smallish strips
1 large bunch parsley, chopped
2/3 cup torn radicchio
2/3 cup chopped curly endive
2/3 cup chopped frizee
3 tomatoes, each cut in 8 lengthwise wedges
1/8 of a large, sweet red onion, thinly sliced
2 tablespoons chopped black olives

Dressing
1/4 cup water
1/2 cup tarragon vinegar
1/2 teaspoon salt or Vege-Sal
1 1/2 tablespoons lemon juice
1 tablespoon Splenda
1/8 teaspoon blackstrap molasses

Topping
6 tablespoons sour cream

1. Put the peppers, parsley, radicchio, endive, frizee, tomatoes, onion, and olives in a big bowl, and set aside.
2. In a separate bowl, combine the water, vinegar, salt, lemon juice, Splenda, and molasses. Pour it allover the salad, and toss.
3. Stick the whole thing in the refrigerator, and let it sit there for a few hours, stirring it now and then if you think of it.
4. To serve, put a 1-tablespoon dollop of sour cream on each serving.

Yield: 6 servings, each with 9 grams of carbohydrates and 2 grams of fiber, for a
total of 7 grams of usable carbs and 2 grams of protein.

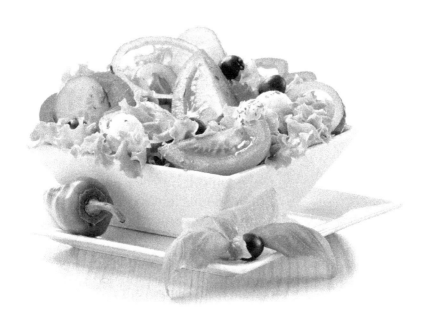

Hot Vegetable Dishes

When folks first go low-carb, they suddenly don't know what to serve for side dishes. The answer is vegetables. If you're used to thinking of vegetables as something that sits between the meat and the potato, usually being ignored, read this chapter and think again!

Here, right up front, are three recipes that every low-carber needs:

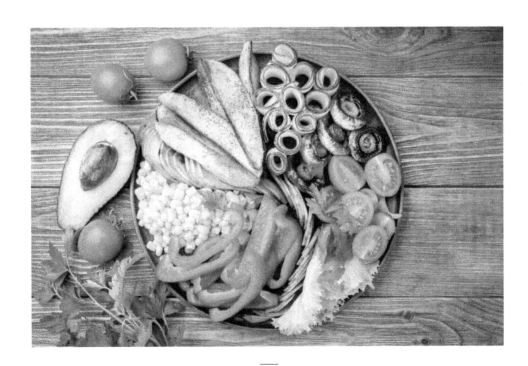

Cauliflower Puree
(a.k.a."Fauxtatoes")

This is a wonderful substitute for mashed potatoes if you want something to put a fabulous sour cream gravy on! Feel free, by the way, touse frozen cauliflower instead; it works quite well here.

1 head fresh or 1 1/2 pounds frozen cauliflower
4 tablespoons butter
Salt and pepper

1. Steam or microwave the cauliflower until it's soft.
2. Drain it thoroughly, and put it through the blender or food processor until it's well pureed. Add the butter and salt and pepper to taste.

Yield: 6 generous servings, each with 5 grams of carbohydrates and 2 grams of fiber, for a total of 3 grams of usable carbs and 2 grams of protein.

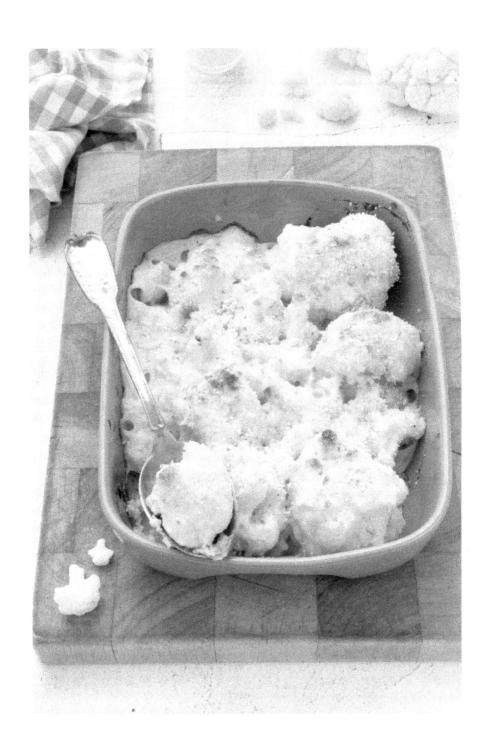

Fauxtatoes Deluxe

This extra-rich fauxtatoes recipe comes from Adele Hite, and it is the basis for the "grits" part of her Low-Carb Shrimp and Grits recipe.

1 large head cauliflower
1/3 cup cream
4 ounces cream cheese
1 tablespoon butter
Salt and pepper

1. Simmer the cauliflower in water with the cream added to it. (This keeps the cauliflower sweet and prevents it from turning an unappetizing gray color.) When the cauliflower is very soft, drain thoroughly.
2. Put the still-warm cauliflower in a food processor with the cream cheese, butter, and salt and pepper to taste, and process until smooth. (You may have to do this in more than one batch.)

Yield: 6 generous servings, each with 6 grams of carbohydrates and 2 grams of fiber, for a total of 4 grams of usable carbs and 4 grams of protein.

~ Give your fauxtatoes a little zing by adding a few cloves of sliced garlic to the cooking water or some roasted garlic to the food processor when blending the cauliflower with the other ingredients. Each clove of garlic added will add just 1 gram of carbohydrates to the carb count for the batch.

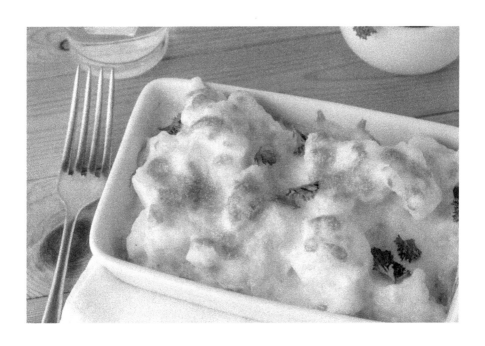

Cauliflower Rice

Many thanks to Fran McCullough! I got this idea from her book Living Carb, and it's served me very well.

1/2 head cauliflower

Simply put the cauliflower through your food processor using the shredding blade. This gives the cauliflower a texture that's remarkably similar to rice. You can steam, microwave, or even saute it in butter. Whatever you do, though, don't overcook it!

Yield: About 3 cups, or 3 servings, each with 5 grams of carbohydrates and 2 grams of fiber, for a total of 3 grams of usable carbs and 2 grams of protein.

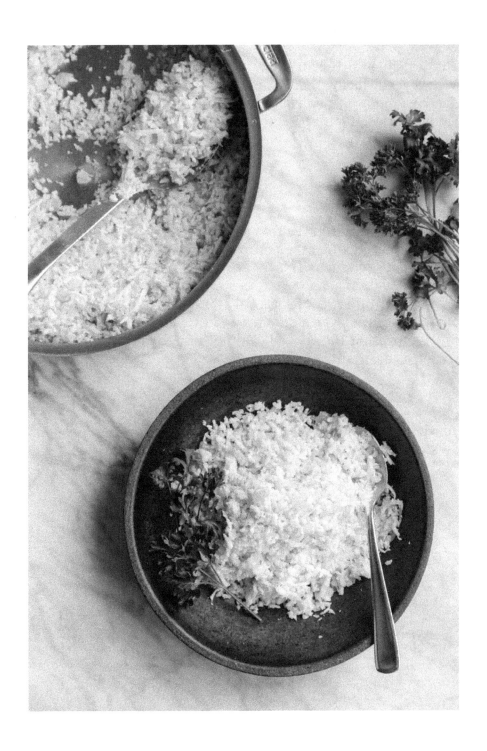

Cauliflower Rice Deluxe

This is higher-carb than plain Cauliflower Rice, but the wild rice adds a grain flavor that makes it quite convincing. Plus, wild rice has about 25 percent less carbohydrates than most other kinds of rice. I only use this for special occasions, but it's wonderful.

3 cups Cauliflower Rice
1/4 cup wild rice
3/4 cup water

1. Cook your cauliflower rice as desired (I steam mine when making this), taking care not to overcook it to mushiness, but just until it's tender.
2. Put the wild rice and water in a saucepan, cover it, and set it on a burner on lowest heat until all the water is gone (at least one-half hour, maybe a bit more).
3. Toss together the cooked cauliflower rice and wild rice, and season as desired.

Yield: 4 cups, or 8 servings, each with 6 grams of carbohydrates and 1 gram of fiber,
for a total of 5 grams of usable carbs and 2 grams of protein.

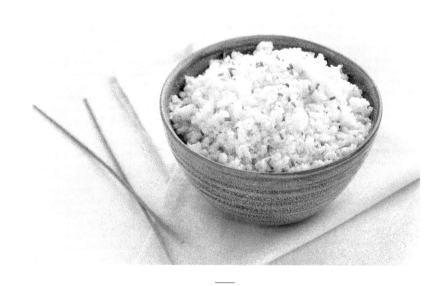

Company Dinner "Rice"

This is my favorite way to season the cauliflower-wild rice blend above. It's a big hit at dinner parties!

1 small onion, chopped
1 stick butter, melted
4 cups Cauliflower Rice Deluxe (see above)
6 strips bacon, cooked until crisp, and crumbled
1/4 teaspoon salt or Vege-Sal
1/4 teaspoon pepper
1/2 cup grated Parmesan cheese

Saute the onion in the butter until it's golden and limp. Toss the Cauliflower Rice Deluxe with the sauteed onion and the bacon, salt, pepper, and cheese. Serve.

Yield: 8 servings, each with 8 grams of carbohydrates and 2 grams of fiber, for a total of 6 grams of usable carbs and 5 grams of protein.

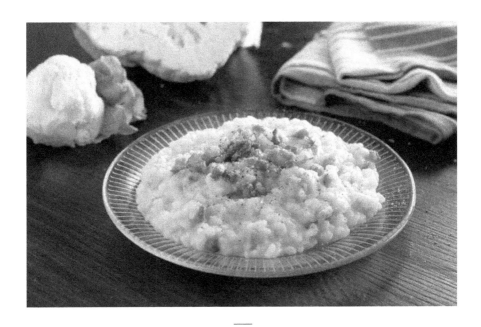

Sauteed Mushrooms

What could be better with a steak? Feel free to play with this recipeuse all butter or all olive oil, throw in a clove of garlic, try a few variations until you find what you like.

2 tablespoons butter
2 tablespoons olive oil
8 ounces mushrooms, thickly sliced
Salt and pepper

1. Melt the butter and heat the olive oil over medium-high heat in a heavy skillet.
2. Add the mushrooms and saute, stirring frequently, for 5 to 7 minutes, or until the mushrooms are limp and brown. Salt and pepper lightly, and serve.

Yield: 3 generous servings, each with 4 grams of carbohydrates and 1 gram of fiber,
for a total of 3 grams of usable carbs and 2 grams of protein.

~ Try this recipe with mushrooms other than the familiar "button" 'shrooms. Criminis and portobellos are both delicious prepared this way, for instance. Avoid shitakes, however; they are much higher in carbohydrates.

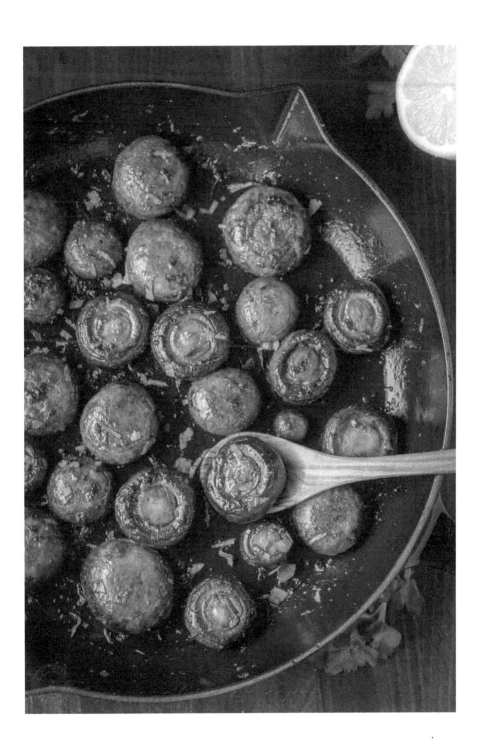

Mushrooms in Sherry Cream

This is rich and flavorful, and best served with a simple roast or the like.

8 ounces small, very fresh mushrooms
1/4 cup dry sherry
1/4 teaspoon salt or Vege-Sal, divided
1/2 cup sour cream
1 clove garlic
1/8 teaspoon pepper

1. Wipe the mushrooms clean, and trim the woody ends off the stems.
2. Place the mushrooms in a small saucepan with the sherry, and sprinkle with 1/8 teaspoon of sa It.
3. Bring the sherry to a boil, turn the burner to low, cover the pan, and let the mushrooms simmer for just 3 to 4 minutes, shaking the pan once or twice while they're cooking.
4. In another saucepan over very low heat, stir together the remaining 1/8 teaspoon salt, sour cream, garlic, and pepper. You want to heat the sour cream through, but don't let it boil, or it will separate.
5. When the mushrooms are done, pour off the liquid into a small bowl. As soon as the sour cream is heated through, spoon it over the mushrooms, and stir everything around over medium-low heat. If it seems a bit thick, add a teaspoon or two of the reserved liquid.
6. Stir the mushrooms and sour cream together for 2 to 3 minutes, again making sure that the sour cream does not boil, and serve.

Yield: 3 servings, each with 4 grams carbohydrates and 1 gram of fiber, for a total of
3 grams of usable carbs and 2 grams of protein.

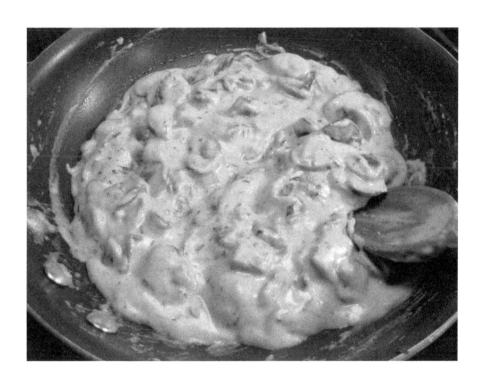

Slice of Mushroom Heaven

Rich enough to give Dean Ornish fits, and oh-so-good. Thanks to my friend Kay for the name!

4 tablespoons butter
1 pound mushrooms, sliced
1/2 medium onion, finely chopped
1 clove garlic, crushed
1/4 cup dry white wine
1 teaspoon lemon juice
1 1/2 cups ha lf -a nd-ha lf
3 eggs
1 teaspoon salt or Vege-Sal
1/4 teaspoon pepper
3 cups shredded Gruyere cheese (a little more than 1/2 pound)

1. Preheat the oven to 350°F.
2. Melt the butter in a heavy skillet over medium heat, and begin frying the mushrooms, onion, and garlic. When the mushrooms are limp, turn the heat up a bit and boil off the liquid. Stir in the white wine, and cook until that's boiled away, too.
3. Stir in the lemon juice and turn off the heat. Transfer the mixture to a large mixing bowl, and stir in the half-and-half, eggs, salt, pepper, and 2 cups of the cheese.
4. Spray an 8 x 8-inch baking pan with nonstick cooking spray, and spread the mixture from step 3 evenly over the bottom. Sprinkle the rest of the cheese on top, and bake for 50 minutes, or until the cheese on top is golden.

*Yield: 9 generous servings, each with 5 grams of carbohydrates and 1 gram of fiber,
for a total of 4 grams of usable carbs and 13 grams of protein.*
~ This dish is good hot, but I actually like it better cold-plus, when it's cold, it cuts in nice, neat squares. I think it makes a nice breakfast or lunch, and
it's definitely a fine side dish. It would even make a good vegetarian main course.

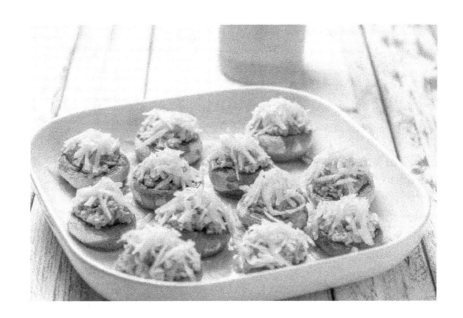

Kolokythia Krokettes

These are rapidly becoming one of our favorite side dishes. They're Greek, and very, very tasty. A terrific side dish with roast lamb or Greek roasted chicken.

3 medium zucchini, grated
1 teaspoon salt or Vege-Sal
3 eggs
1 cup crumbled feta
1 teaspoon dried oregano
1/2 medium onion, finely diced
1/8 teaspoon pepper
3 tablespoons soy powder or rice protein powder
Butter

~ Shave some time preparing the ingredients for this dish by running the zucchini and the onion through a food processor.

1. Mix the grated zucchini with the salt in a bowl, and let it sit for an hour or so. Squeeze out and drain the liquid.
2. Mix in the eggs, feta, oregano, onion, pepper, and soy powder, and combine well.
3. Spray a heavy skillet with nonstick cooking spray, add a healthy tablespoon of butter, and melt over medium heat. Fry the batter by the tablespoonful, turning once. Add more butter between batches, as needed, and keep the cooked krokettes warm. The trick to these is to let them get quite brown on the bottom before trying to turn them, or they tend to fall apart. If a few do fall apart, don't sweat it; the pieces will still taste incredible.

Yield: 6 servings, each with 6 grams of carbohydrates and 2 grams of fiber, for a
total of 4 grams usable carbs and 8 grams of protein.

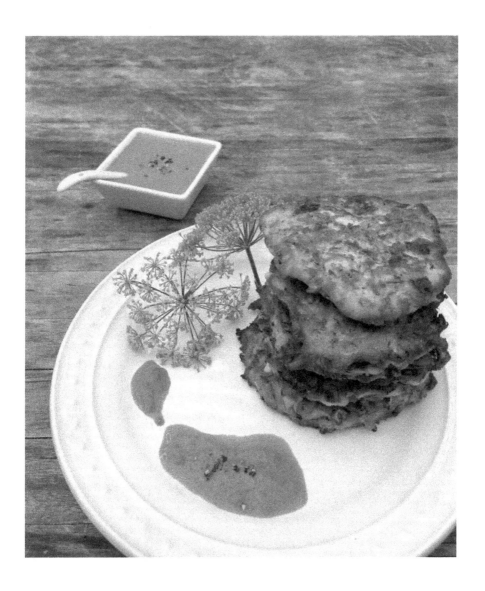

Zucchini With Sour Cream

For People Who Don't Love Zucchini Marilee Wellersdick sends this recipe. My sister, who tested it, says the name is no joke-it went over well with nonzucchini-loving in-laws.

4 tablespoons butter
1 medium onion, chopped
8 small zucchini, sliced about 1/8 inch thick
Salt and pepper
1 cup sour cream

1. Melt the butter in a large, preferably nonstick skillet. Add the onion and zucchini, and salt and pepper to taste.
2. Cover and cook on medium heat, stirring occasionally, until the zucchini is translucent (15 to 20 minutes).
3. Remove from the heat, and stir in the sour cream. Serve.

Yield: 6 servings, each with 11 grams of carbohydrates and 3 grams of fiber, for a
total of 8 grams of usable carbs and no protein.

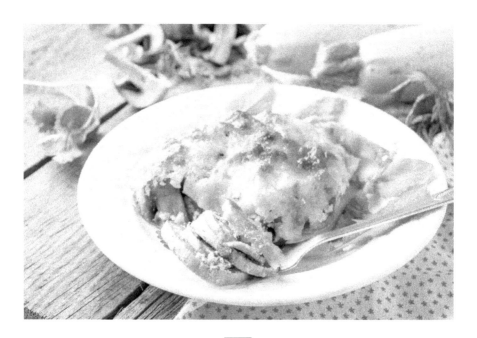

Zucchini Casserole

Jodee Rushton, who contributed this recipe, says, "Since each serving has protein as well as vegetable, it's great as part of a lunch with some other veggies. It's also a great snack."

2 tablespoons butter
1 1/2 pounds zucchini, unpeeled, washed, and sliced
2 eggs, beaten
1 tablespoon unbleached flour
1/2 teaspoon dry mustard
1/2 teaspoon ground nutmeg
1/2 teaspoon salt
Pepper
1 packet Splenda
1 cup heavy cream
6 ounces sharp Cheddar cheese, shredded

1. Preheat the oven to 325°F, and spray a large casserole with nonstick cooking spray.
2. Melt the butter in a large, heavy skillet. Add the sliced zucchini, and saute over medium-high heat until tender, stirring frequently. When done, remove from the heat and let cool until lukewarm. Place in the prepared casserole.
3. Combine the eggs, flour, mustard, nutmeg, salt, pepper to taste, and Splenda in a large mixing bowl; whisk together well. Add the heavy cream and Cheddar, and mix well.
4. Add the egg mixture to the cooled zucchini, and mix well. Place in the oven, and bake for 30 minutes or until set. Cool and serve.

*Yield: 6 servings, each with 6 grams of carbohydrates and 1 gram of fiber, for a total
of 5 grams of usable carbs and 11 grams of protein.*

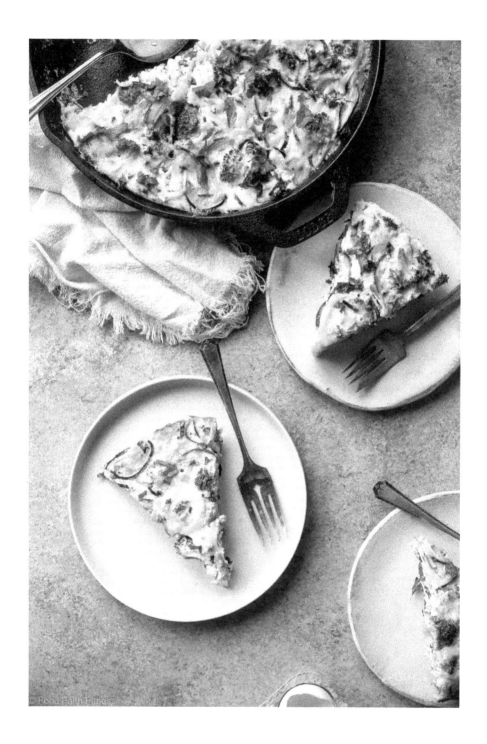

Zucchini-Crusted Pizza

This is like a somewhat-mare-substantial quiche on the bottom, and pizza on top.

3 1/2 cups shredded zucchini
3 eggs
1/3 cup rice protein powder or soy powder
1 1/2 cups shredded mozzarella
1/2 cup grated Parmesan cheese
A pi nch or two of dried basi I
1/2 teaspoon salt
1/4 teaspoon pepper
Oil
1 cup sugarless pizza sauce
Toppings as desired (sausage, pepperoni, peppers, mushrooms,
or whatever you like)

1. Preheat the oven to 350°F.
2. Sprinkle the zucchini with a little salt, and let it sit for 15 to 30 minutes. Put it in a strainer and press out the excess moisture.
3. Beat together the strained zucchini, eggs, protein powder, 1/2 cup of mozzarella, Parmesan, basil, salt, and pepper.
4. Spray a 9 x 13-inch baking pan with nonstick cooking spray, and spread the zucchini mixture in it.
5. Bake for about 25 minutes, or until firm. Brush it with a little oil, and broil it for about 5 minutes, until it's golden.
6. Next, spread on the pizza sauce, then add the remaining 1 cup of mozzarella and other toppings.
7. Bake for another 25 minutes, then cut into squares and serve.

Yield: 4 generous servings, each with 14 grams of carbohydrates and 2 grams of fiber, for a total of 12 grams of usable carbs and 22 grams of protein. (Analysis does not include toppings.)

———

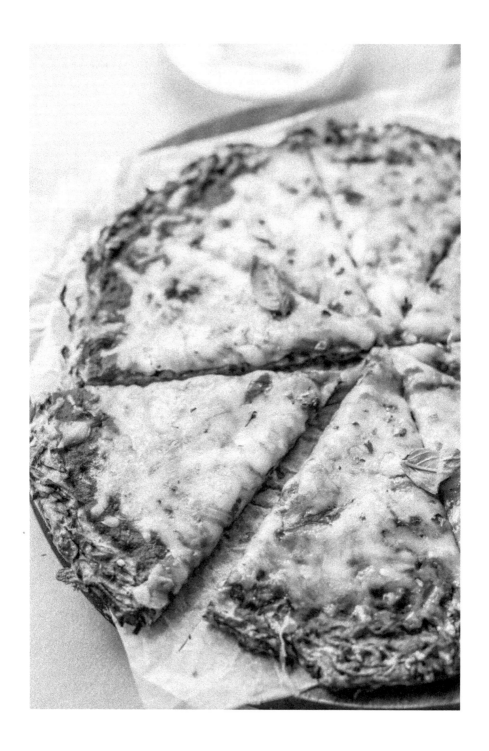

Eggplant Parmesan Squared

When you use Parmesan cheese instead of breadcrumbs to "bread" the eggplant slices, it becomes Eggplant Parmesan Squared! This takes a little doing, but it's delicious, and it's easily filling enough for a main dish.

1/2 cup low-carb bake mix or unflavored protein powder
2 or 3 eggs ~
1 1/4 to 1 3/4 cups Parmesan cheese ~
1 large eggplant, sliced no more than 1/4-inch thick
Olive oil for frying
1 clove garlic, cut in half
1 1/2 cups sugar-free spaghetti sauce
8 ounces shredded mozzarella

~ How many eggs and how much cheese you will need depends on how big your eggplant is.

1. Preheat the oven to 350°F.
2. Put the bake mix on a plate, break the eggs into a shallow bowl and beat well, and put 1 to 1 1/2 cups of Parmesan on another plate.
3. Dip each eggplant slice in the bake mix so each side is well dusted.
4. Dip each "floured" slice of eggplant in the beaten egg and then in the Parmesan so that each slice has a good coating of the cheese. Refrigerate the "breaded" slices of eggplant for at least half an hour, or up to an hour or two.
5. Pour 1/8 inch of olive oil in the bottom of a heavy skillet over medium heat. Add the garlic, letting it sizzle for a minute or two before removing. Now fry the refrigerated eggplant slices until they're golden brown on both sides (you 'll have to add more olive oil as you go along.)
6. Spread 1/2 cup of spaghetti sauce in the bottom of a 9 x 11-inch roasting pan.

Arrange half of the eggplant slices to cover bottom of pan. Cover with the mozzarella, and top with the remaining eggplant. Pour the rest of the spaghetti sauce on, and sprinkle the remaining 1/4 cup of Parmesan on top.

7. Bake for 30 minutes.

Yield: 6 servings, each with 13 grams of carbohydrates and 4.5 grams of fiber, for a total of 8.5 usable carbs and 24 grams of protein.

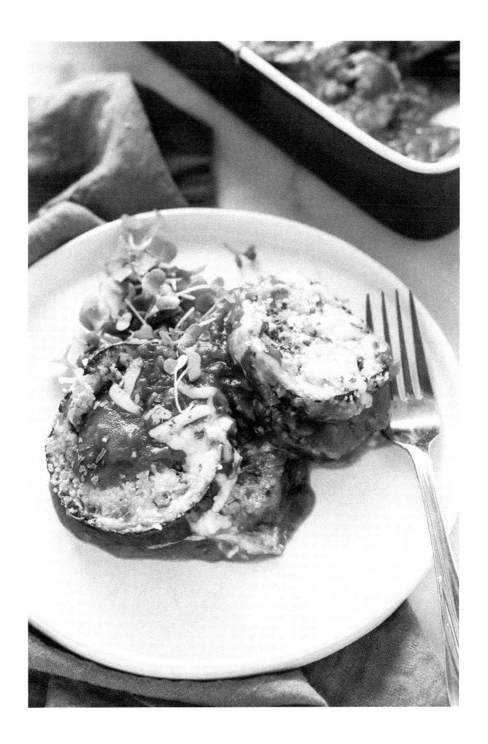

CPSIA information can be obtained
at www.ICGtesting.com
Printed in the USA
BVHW081156140521
607268BV00002B/450